The Complete Guide to Digestive Health

Plain Answers about IBS, Constipation, Diarrhea, Heartburn, Ulcers, and More

Publisher's Note

The editors of FC&A have taken careful measures to ensure the accuracy and usefulness of the information in this book. While every attempt was made to assure accuracy, some Web sites, addresses, telephone numbers, and other information may have changed since printing.

This book is intended for general information only. It does not constitute medical advice or practice. We cannot guarantee the safety or effectiveness of any treatment or advice mentioned. Readers are urged to consult with their health care professionals and get their approval before undertaking therapies suggested by information in this book, keeping in mind that errors in the text may occur as in all publications and that new findings may supercede older information.

> *"And all the people were trying to touch Him, for power was coming from Him and healing them all."*
>
> *Luke 6:19*

Contents

CHAPTER 4

Best bets for better digestion 163

CHAPTER 5

Diet additions to aid digestion 195

CHAPTER 6

Products and therapies: What you should know

CHAPTER 7

Medical tests to diagnose digestive diseases 329

An amazing personal story: Can sulforaphane in broccoli products help heal digestive problems?

Several months ago, my two sons experienced severe digestive problems while away at college. First one and then the other began to suffer intermittent abdominal pain and diarrhea that became increasingly severe over several months. One was losing weight, and they both looked and felt sick. One night, my older son had to go to the hospital emergency room after experiencing severe pain in his lower right abdomen, possibly appendicitis. But he was released the next day after the pain went away.

These and other serious symptoms were suggestive of early stage Crohn's disease because of the severity of their illness and a history of inflammatory bowel disease in a close relative. However, Crohn's disease usually is not diagnosed until it has been present for years and there is evidence of severe damage to the bowel. In its early stages, a more generalized diagnosis of IBS may be given to some people who later are determined to have been suffering from Crohn's. In answer to my family's heartfelt prayers, amazing, new information came to light. According to recent research, broccoli products can help heal chronic gastritis caused by infection with the *Helicobacter pylori* bacterium. What's more, many cases of Crohn's disease are thought to be triggered by a run-away immune system reaction to infection with a different bacterium, *Mycobacterium avium paratuberculosis* (MAP) that can hide undetected in the tissues of the intestines.

Realizing that sulforaphane, the newly discovered natural medicine in broccoli, was shown in scientific studies to stimulate the body's production of Phase II enzymes that help attack disease-producing bacteria in a narrowly focused way, without causing unnecessary inflammatory reactions, the thought occurred to me — could sulforaphane, that acts as a natural antibiotic and immune system regulator, stimulate the body to kill MAP bacteria and also help dampen the run-away immune system reaction that causes Crohn's disease? Excited by the possibility, I talked with my sons, and we decided it was worth a try.

Young men off at college are the least likely prospects to try a diet different from regular dorm food or pizza. But things were so bad they were willing to try anything. Their "treatment" was nothing more than eating 2 ounces — about one cup — of broccoli sprouts every day. The seeds and sprouts of broccoli contain several times as much sulforaphane as stalks and florets. Later, for convenience, the boys substituted a teaspoon of broccoli seeds a day when they ran out of sprouts. (Not many college students living in dorms are into "sprouting.") These small amounts of broccoli sprouts or seeds were enough to provide a sufficient therapeutic amount of sulforaphane, according to research studies.

Both of my sons started feeling better within one week of eating broccoli sprouts or seeds daily. Within two months, my youngest son, who had less-severe symptoms, was almost fully recovered. After the third month, his older brother was free of the worst symptoms, although he still has occasional heartburn. (Crohn's disease may sometimes damage the esophagus, as well as other parts of the digestive tract.) Heartburn, or gastroesophageal reflux, is easily controlled with an acid reducer. Occasional heartburn is a relatively minor problem for him compared to the horrible pain and other distressing symptoms of his illness.

My sons now need little prompting to continue eating broccoli products two to four days per week. The only hint of a reoccurrence of major symptoms occurred after my youngest son, thinking he was fully cured, neglected to eat his broccoli products for a few weeks. Does this amazing story prove that sulforaphane in broccoli can help heal IBS or Crohn's disease? By no means — not until confirmed by scientific studies. But this experience does suggest a dietary approach that could prove to be very helpful. Eating broccoli products is a food therapy that can be tried without discarding other treatments or ignoring medical advice. Ask your doctor if he thinks it's worth a try.

Additional information can be found in the *Broccoli sprouts*, *Tea*, *Irritable bowel syndrome*, *Gastritis*, and *Crohn's disease* chapters in this book. For more information about the discovery of sulforaphane in broccoli, see page 60 of the January/February 2004 issue of *The Saturday Evening Post.*

Frank K. Wood

YOU'RE NOT ALONE IF YOU FACE
PROBLEMS WITH YOUR DIGESTIVE
SYSTEM. Sales of digestive remedies
reached more than $2.5 billion in
2004, and the National Institute of
Diabetes and Digestive and Kidney
Diseases reports that digestive dis-
eases affect at least 60 million people.

CHAPTER 1

Why people get digestive diseases

Every day scientists and doctors
around the world determinedly hunt
new ways to fight digestive problems. And many people who have
the same digestive illness trade tips
and information to help each other.
Some meet in local support groups,
while others take advantage of the
Internet's worldwide reach.

Celebrities now speak out about their fights with unglamorous conditions, like inflammatory bowel disease. They hope to help others find answers more quickly.

These people wield knowledge as their weapon against digestive distress, and you can, too. Get a head start on getting better. Review how your digestive system works, uncover common trouble triggers, and find out about scientific theories and discoveries that might help you.

Take a cruise down the alimentary canal

Remember how the submarine in *Fantastic Voyage* could travel throughout the human body? You could easily navigate a miniature submarine through the entire digestive system because the GI tract is a tunnel of hollow organs linked together. Fortunately, you don't need a submarine. Your VIP tour of the digestive system, through the alimentary canal, starts right now, and you won't even have to leave your chair.

The first stop on the tour is your mouth. This is the first place you'll see the protective inner lining called the mucosa. Nearly all the digestive organs have this remarkable lining. The mouth is also the place where the GI tract's chemical wizardry begins. For example, an enzyme in saliva helps digest the starch from food into smaller molecules.

When health professionals talk about the digestive system, you may hear terms like gastrointestinal tract, alimentary canal, GI tract, or gut.

Proper chewing breaks down food to just the right size and consistency to go down the throat. Enzymes in saliva help break down food and begin digestion. Other factors in saliva help protect the lining of the digestive tract as saliva lubricates the passage of food to the stomach. When the tongue pushes food back and triggers the swallowing reflex, the voice box closes and breathing stops for a moment so food stays out of your windpipe. Then, the food starts down the esophagus — the next stop on the tour.

The esophagus is a 10-inch tube that delivers food to the stomach. Its muscular walls usher food along with a distinctive motion called peristalsis. Peristalsis rolls down the esophagus like an ocean wave. The muscles make a segment at the top of the esophagus constrict, and then send this wave of constriction slowly down the length of the esophagus. More peristalsis waves follow — just like waves at the seashore. These waves move food and fluid ahead of them through the esophagus with incredible smoothness, yet they're so strong that you can even swallow while you're upside down.

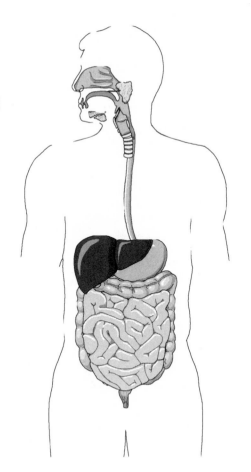

A helpful ring-shaped valve, called the lower esophageal sphincter, guards the bottom end of the esophagus. It usually keeps the doorway between the esophagus and the stomach closed. But, when food arrives, it relaxes temporarily to let the food enter the stomach. Then it contracts again to keep the stomach's contents from sneaking back into the esophagus.

The next stop on the tour is the stomach. Located in the upper abdomen, it resembles a stretchy sack. In fact, it can stretch out to hold about three pints. How? The muscle of the upper part of the stomach relaxes to make extra room.

Meanwhile, the lower part of the stomach uses heavy-duty muscle action to mix food and liquid with digestive juices. Tiny glands in the stomach lining supply juices, like protein-digesting enzymes and high-powered stomach acid that's important for killing bacteria while helping digest food.

Peristalsis also helps move food through other parts of the digestive tract.

Stomach acid is corrosive enough to dissolve food, so it could easily damage the stomach or any other organ. But, in most people, sufficient mucus from the stomach's mucous membranes coats the lining of the stomach and resists the acid so the stomach tissue is protected.

When the stomach has thoroughly mixed the food with digestive juices, it gradually empties its contents into the small intestine.

The small intestine can take a while to tour. If you could stretch out all its twists and turns, the small intestine would be a spectacular 20-feet long. Incredibly, fine hair-like projections called villi cover the small intestine walls. They help absorb nutrients into the bloodstream.

After the stomach empties into the small intestine, digestive juices from the pancreas and liver mix with the food.

▸ The pancreas secretes digestive enzymes through a tube called the pancreatic duct. These enzymes don't become active until they reach the small intestine. Then they team up with vital enzymes from the small intestine lining to help digest fats, proteins, and carbohydrates.

▸ The liver produces a digestive juice called bile and stores it in the gallbladder. At mealtime, especially a meal that includes fat, bile passes through the bile ducts and on to the small intestine. Like grease-busting dish detergent, bile dissolves fat into the watery contents of the intestine.

The small intestine has three sections, starting with the duodenum. The last two parts, the jejunum and ileum, absorb digested molecules of food, water, vitamins, and miner-als. Most absorbed nutrients cross the mucosa into the bloodstream.

After the intestinal walls filter out all the digested nutrients, only waste products are left. These include water and undigested parts of food, known as "fiber," which has now become mush.

Enzymes from the small intestine lining are impor-tant because you need them to digest carbohy-drates like lactose — the sugar in milk — and table sugar. Other small intestine enzymes help split proteins into nutritious amino acids.

The last attraction of the tour, the colon or large intestine, is around 5 feet long. It starts with the vertical "ascending" colon on the right side followed by the horizontal transverse colon, the descending colon on the left, and the S-shaped sigmoid colon, which leads to the anus with its circular anal sphincter muscles. The colon removes water from the waste as it passes through. This usually takes a day or two. Then the waste is removed by a bowel movement.

But that's not all that happens in the colon. Although a newborn baby's colon doesn't have any naturally occurring microbes, every-one's colon gains hundreds of kinds of bacteria and other microorganisms early in life. These are called "intestinal flora." Some of these microorganisms can cause disease, but most of them help keep you healthy. The "good" bacteria like to grow in the presence of mushy soluble fiber. The "bad" bacteria like a fiber-depleted environ-ment. Some of these tiny allies make substances that inhibit the growth of harmful fungi and bacteria. Others may help your body make vitamin K or unleash anti-inflammatory powers. Good bacteria even secrete enzymes that help digestion.

Discover your gut's miraculous partners

Your GI tract doesn't work alone, but you may be surprised to find out who its close partners are — your nervous system and immune system.

Your GI tract includes around 100 million nerve cells. That's almost as many nerve cells as your whole spinal cord. In fact, your digestive tract constantly trades information with your central nervous system.

Like other parts of your body, your digestive system is sprinkled with dense masses of nerve cells called ganglia. But, while ganglia from other parts of the body are just designed to relay information from the brain, GI ganglia sport a different framework and chemical make-up. They can help the digestive system tackle some problems without the brain. Perhaps that's why scientists refer to all those nerve cells in the gut as the enteric nervous system or the "brain-in-the-gut."

The walls of the esophagus, stomach, small intestine, and colon all contain a dense network of nerves. When food stretches the walls of an organ, these nerves leap into action. They can release many different substances to speed up or slow down the movement of food and production of digestive juices in the organ they control.

> The small intestine is about four times as long as the large intestine. So why is the large intestine called large? Because it has a wider diameter than the small intestine.

Nerves also come into the digestive organs from the brain or spinal cord. The nerves release messenger chemicals called acetylcholine and adrenaline. Acetylcholine causes the muscles of the digestive organs to propel food through the GI tract with more force. Adrenaline relaxes the stomach and intestinal muscles and reduces blood flow to these organs.

With all these links between the brain and the GI tract, it's no wonder that researchers are testing how well stress busters may combat digestive disorders.

But your GI tract has another surprise. As much as 80 percent of your body's immune cells live in your digestive system. That may sound strange, but remember — you can get a "stomach virus" from something you eat. If your immune system's job is to turn your body into a fortress against outside invaders, it must guard key entry-ways, like your digestive system. So the immune system puts defenders along the GI tract walls.

Your stomach acid destroys many troublemaking microbes swallowed with food. Microbes that survive that front-line defense still have to battle through the walls of the digestive tract to the underlying cells.

That's no easy task because the mucosa — the digestive tract lining — is shielded by protective mucus and more. So if a harmful microbe doesn't get trapped in the mucous coating, it may still be blocked by the tightly packed cells in the mucosa's top layer. And lurking beneath that is the gut-associated lymphoid tissue or GALT. This is where many types of immune cells lie in wait for any germ that makes it through the mucosa. As long as this immune defense system continues to work properly, most microbes don't stand a chance.

In fact, your entire digestive system does a great job as long as it runs properly, but you need to know why it stops working as it should.

Outsmart these menacing villains

Many villains can keep your digestive system from working perfectly, but the "most wanted" often come from this list.

▸ harmful bacteria

▸ immune problems and inflammation

▸ family history

▸ lifestyle factors, like diet, weight, medication, stress, or health habits

It's no surprise that viruses and bacteria can cause food poisoning and traveler's diarrhea. But scientists were surprised to learn that most ulcers, and many cases of chronic upset stomach, or gastritis, are caused by *Helicobacter pylori* (*H. pylori*) bacteria and can be cured by antibiotics. Now scientists say that most people who get stomach cancer are infected with *H. pylori*. So eliminating the bacteria should lower your risk of stomach cancer, but eliminating *H. pylori* may be a double-edged sword. The presence of certain relatively benign strains of *H. pylori* residing in the stomach may help to regulate stomach acid levels without greatly increasing rates of stomach cancer.

Some researchers also think certain types of bacteria — especially *Mycobacterium avium paratuberculosis* or MAP — may contribute to Crohn's disease. In fact, MAP may infect cows and pass to you through their milk.

Meanwhile, scientists suspect that keeping enough probiotic, or friendly, bacteria in your system may help lower your risk of colon cancer and inflammatory bowel disease.

Exciting new theories suggest inflammation and immune problems may also hold clues to digestive mysteries.

Powerful help for your immune system

Inflammatory bowel disease, allergies, and several other conditions seem to be on the rise in modern Western countries and in other places with widespread good hygiene habits. These diseases all have one thing in common — an out-of-control immune reaction.

The hygiene hypothesis suggests why this might happen. Although you have many types of immune cells, this hypothesis focuses on white blood cells called Th1 and Th2. Th1 cells attack infected cells throughout your body. Th2 cells produce antibodies to block dangerous microbes from invading your body's cells in the first place, but if they are too active, they may also trigger allergic reactions, including reactions in the digestive tract.

Th1 and Th2 should balance out each other to keep you healthy. But, according to the hygiene hypothesis, Th1 cells aren't strong enough to defend you right after you're born — only Th2 cells are. This hypothesis also suggests that Th1 cells can only get up to full strength by fighting off infections or interacting with certain soil microbes. But if modern hygiene keeps you away from microbes and infections, perhaps Th1 cells stay too weak to keep Th2 cells under control. And Th2 cells gone amuck may lead to high rates of allergies and inflammatory bowel disease.

But, oddly enough, some conditions may be caused by Th1 cells raging out of control instead of Th2 cells — and these conditions are on the increase in nations with super-clean hygiene, as well. That's where a third group of immune cells — called T-regulators — may come in. Some scientists suggest that people who grow up in less-hygienic environments than most Americans have greater exposure to parasites, such as pig whipworms or soil microbes, and this exposure enables T-regulators to keep both Th1 and Th2 cells in bounds.

Like any new study or theory that contradicts past research, the hygiene hypothesis will require much more testing to find out whether it's true. So stay tuned for more research results. And before you try treatment based on this theory, discuss the research and proposed treatment with your doctor.

Inflammation might be the root of many diseases

Like bad-tasting medicine that helps make you better, inflammation is meant to be a good thing. All that redness and swelling is a perfectly normal body response to a cut on your finger or an infection. Inflammation helps fend off viruses and other microbe-size invaders. It also stays just long enough to prepare the way for healing after an injury or illness — but once in awhile something goes wrong.

Scientists have already linked several diseases with inflammation, including Crohn's disease, ulcers, and cancer. But the "inflammation theory" suggests that many more diseases may be linked with inflammation that either goes haywire or simply doesn't quit when it should.

For example, chronic inflammation might encourage tumors to grow and spread. The theory is that tumors, which look like wounds to your body, promote inflammation, and inflammatory cells encourage cell growth — even for cancer cells. That might mean anti-inflammatory therapies could help slow the disease.

Scientists are studying whether inflammation may cause or aggravate other conditions, so keep an eye out for more exciting results.

Make amazing enzymes work for you

Your body has special enzymes and substances assigned to help take out nonfunctional cells or cancer-causing garbage that sneaks in. Some of these special enzymes are called phase II detoxification enzymes. Phase II enzymes are more specifically targeted to what's wrong than the other parts of the immune system that can go into overdrive and cause excessive inflammation. Not only do they help inactivate cancer-causing substances, phase II enzymes also repackage them so your body can get rid of them more quickly — like bagging up trash so it's easier to take to the curb.

Perhaps the best part about phase II enzymes is that you can get more of them working for you. Broccoli and other cruciferous vegetables contain compounds, like sulforaphane, that boost these cancer-busting enzymes so your body won't forget to take out the trash. They might even help to get rid of bad bacteria that may cause digestive problems.

Do a background check on yourself

You can't look into the future to find out whether you'll develop GI problems, but looking into the past might help. That's because a high risk of a particular GI problem could be in your genes. And finding out could help you take steps to prevent it or solve the mystery of what's ailing you.

First, check your family history. You're more likely to develop colon cancer if someone in your immediate family has also had it.

If your family history is clean, consider where your ancestors came from. People with Scandinavian ancestry are more likely to get gallstones, while those with African or Asian ancestry have a higher risk of lactose intolerance. And people with European, especially European-Jewish, ancestors are more prone to get Crohn's disease.

Shift the odds in your favor

You may be surprised at how much you can help yourself if you're at risk for a GI problem or even if you already have one.

What you put into your digestive system can make a difference. Good eating leads to good digesting. So dig into a health-promoting diet and avoid foods that trigger your symptoms. Start with these guidelines.

> ▸ **Find out the trigger foods** for your symptoms or condition. Heartburn, gas, diarrhea, ulcerative colitis, celiac disease, irritable bowel syndrome, Crohn's disease, and food allergies are examples of conditions where particular foods or food groups can trigger a flare-up or make things worse.

> ▸ **Aim for nine delicious servings** of fruits and vegetables every day. Eating more of these and less red meat can help guard you against heartburn, constipation, and more.

> ▸ **Trade that wimpy white bread** for heartier whole-grain goodness. Sugar, white flour, and other highly processed starches may lead to stomachache and boost cancer risk.

> ▸ **Eat whole-grain cereals,** breads, and snacks and drink plenty of water. You may find that whole grains help prevent constipation and many other ills, while the water helps prevent bloating and gas that extra fiber can bring.

> ▸ **Get plenty of calcium** from green leafy vegetables, fortified cereals, and — if you can tolerate it — low-fat dairy foods.

> ▸ **Limit the fat in your diet,** and you could thwart heartburn, painful IBS symptoms, and more — while cutting your risk of serious conditions. Trade the saturated fats and trans fats of packaged foods and red meats for the healthier fats in nuts, seeds, and fish.

> ▸ **Avoid fried** or greasy foods.

▸ **Curb your sweet tooth.** Sugary drinks and snacks, even if they only contain artificial sweeteners, can mean gas, diarrhea, or worse for some people.

▸ **Try eliminating coffee** to see if it helps. It's a known trigger for some symptoms and disease flare-ups. So are alcohol and tobacco.

If you're overweight, losing extra pounds might help relieve heartburn. It may also slice your risk of hiatal hernia, gallstones, hemorrhoids, and colon cancer. And if you choose exercise to help you shed weight, you may get a bonus. Exercise may help prevent gas, while slashing your risk of colon cancer and ulcers. Walk, do yardwork, dance, or play a sport. It all counts toward your goal of staying healthy.

Frequent use of nonsteroidal anti-inflammatory drugs (NSAIDs), such as aspirin and ibuprofen, can fuel gastritis and lead to ulcers. They may trigger or aggravate other digestive problems, as well. But NSAIDs may be necessary for some people. Talk with your doctor to find out what's right for you.

Constipation, heartburn, nausea, diarrhea, indigestion, and gas are all known side effects of various over-the-counter or prescription drugs. Ask your doctor or pharmacist whether your digestive symptoms could be caused by medication you take.

Stress can trigger some digestive problems and make others worse. Find ways to manage stress and you may find relief.

This is only the beginning of what you can do to help yourself win against digestive distress. Keep reading for more exciting information.

HEARTBURN, INDIGESTION, GAS, DIARRHEA — most people think of these as illnesses. In fact, they are symptoms of many digestive disorders. They are your body's warning signs of a larger problem. Diarrhea, for instance, has many potential causes, from viral infections to diverticulosis. The same goes for dyspepsia, or indigestion, that unpleasant burning, bloating, gassy, or achy feeling you sometimes get after a big meal.

CHAPTER 2

Symptoms, solutions, and when to seek help

The following pages list some of the most common digestive symptoms. Look up your symptoms to learn what could be causing them, when you should see your doctor, and what you can do at home to relieve the discomfort.

Heartburn

Heartburn is a symptom of acid reflux, or acid indigestion, and the feeling is unmistakable — an uncomfortable burning behind your breastbone that radiates up into your throat and neck. You may even feel food or liquid come up your throat, or get a sour, bitter taste in your mouth.

Common causes. The stomach secretes hydrochloric acid and other juices to digest food. When you eat, food travels down your esophagus into your stomach. A valve at the top of your stomach called the lower esophageal sphincter (LES) relaxes to let the food in, then closes to seal out stomach acid.

But sometimes the LES relaxes at the wrong time, letting stomach acid creep up into your esophagus. That's when the burn begins. Anyone can experience heartburn, but it tends to strike people who are elderly, overweight, or pregnant, especially right after meals or during times of stress. These seven culprits increase your chance of getting heartburn.

- overeating
- obesity
- a weak LES muscle
- hiatal hernia
- eating chocolate or alcohol, which prompts the LES to relax
- wearing tight belts or clothing, which put pressure on the stomach
- some prescription medicines, such as nitrates, calcium channel blockers, and anticholinergics

When to seek help. Occasional heartburn doesn't really hurt you, but chronic heartburn can. If you get it two or more times a week, it's time to see your doctor. Chronic heartburn is called GERD — gastroesophageal reflux disease. Your doctor needs to find out why it's happening before it

2008

For by grace you have been saved through faith; and that not of yourselves, it is the gift of God; not as a result of works, that no one should boast. **Eph. 2:8-9**

JANUARY
```
 S  M  T  W  T  F  S
       1  2  3  4  5
 6  7  8  9 10 11 12
13 14 15 16 17 18 19
20 21 22 23 24 25 26
27 28 29 30 31
```

FEBRUARY
```
 S  M  T  W  T  F  S
                1  2
 3  4  5  6  7  8  9
10 11 12 13 14 15 16
17 18 19 20 21 22 23
24 25 26 27 28 29
```

MARCH
```
 S  M  T  W  T  F  S
                   1
 2  3  4  5  6  7  8
 9 10 11 12 13 14 15
16 17 18 19 20 21 22
23/30 24/31 25 26 27 28 29
```

APRIL
```
 S  M  T  W  T  F  S
       1  2  3  4  5
 6  7  8  9 10 11 12
13 14 15 16 17 18 19
20 21 22 23 24 25 26
27 28 29 30
```

MAY
```
 S  M  T  W  T  F  S
          1  2  3
 4  5  6  7  8  9 10
11 12 13 14 15 16 17
18 19 20 21 22 23 24
25 26 27 28 29 30 31
```

JUNE
```
 S  M  T  W  T  F  S
 1  2  3  4  5  6  7
 8  9 10 11 12 13 14
15 16 17 18 19 20 21
22 23 24 25 26 27 28
29 30
```

JULY
```
 S  M  T  W  T  F  S
       1  2  3  4  5
 6  7  8  9 10 11 12
13 14 15 16 17 18 19
20 21 22 23 24 25 26
27 28 29 30 31
```

AUGUST
```
 S  M  T  W  T  F  S
                1  2
 3  4  5  6  7  8  9
10 11 12 13 14 15 16
17 18 19 20 21 22 23
24/31 25 26 27 28 29 30
```

SEPTEMBER
```
 S  M  T  W  T  F  S
    1  2  3  4  5  6
 7  8  9 10 11 12 13
14 15 16 17 18 19 20
21 22 23 24 25 26 27
28 29 30
```

OCTOBER
```
 S  M  T  W  T  F  S
          1  2  3  4
 5  6  7  8  9 10 11
12 13 14 15 16 17 18
19 20 21 22 23 24 25
26 27 28 29 30 31
```

NOVEMBER
```
 S  M  T  W  T  F  S
                   1
 2  3  4  5  6  7  8
 9 10 11 12 13 14 15
16 17 18 19 20 21 22
23/30 24 25 26 27 28 29
```

DECEMBER
```
 S  M  T  W  T  F  S
    1  2  3  4  5  6
 7  8  9 10 11 12 13
14 15 16 17 18 19 20
21 22 23 24 25 26 27
28 29 30 31
```

Heart attack symptoms go beyond heartburn. If your chest pain includes one or more of the following, forget the antacids and call for emergency help to take you to the hospital.

▸ pain or pressure that lasts longer than a few minutes and radiates from your chest to your shoulder, arm, or jaw — especially on your left side

▸ shortness of breath, cold sweat, nausea, or light-headedness

▸ heart palpitations, fatigue, or anxiety

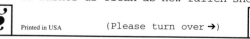

Thank You!

Thank you for being our customer. Your satisfaction is always guaranteed.

I'm sending you this little calendar card as a small token of thanks. I'd also like to show my appreciation by telling you how to have something of far greater value ... a gift more precious than diamonds or gold. This gift is true love, joy, peace and life beyond the grave. It's yours by turning away from sin and following Jesus Christ.

- ▸ He gives us hope when there is none.
- ▸ He gives us life when our candle burns short.
- ▸ He gives us peace when our world is in turmoil.
- ▸ He gives us strength when we are weak.
- ▸ He loves us when no one cares.
- ▸ He washes us clean as new fallen snow.

Printed in USA

(Please turn over ➔)

FCC-08/09

2009

For by grace you have been saved through faith; and that not of yourselves, it is the gift of God; not as a result of works, that no one should boast. **Eph. 2:8-9**

JANUARY
```
 S  M  T  W  T  F  S
             1  2  3
 4  5  6  7  8  9 10
11 12 13 14 15 16 17
18 19 20 21 22 23 24
25 26 27 28 29 30 31
```

FEBRUARY
```
 S  M  T  W  T  F  S
 1  2  3  4  5  6  7
 8  9 10 11 12 13 14
15 16 17 18 19 20 21
22 23 24 25 26 27 28
```

MARCH
```
 S  M  T  W  T  F  S
 1  2  3  4  5  6  7
 8  9 10 11 12 13 14
15 16 17 18 19 20 21
22 23 24 25 26 27 28
29 30 31
```

APRIL
```
 S  M  T  W  T  F  S
          1  2  3  4
 5  6  7  8  9 10 11
12 13 14 15 16 17 18
19 20 21 22 23 24 25
26 27 28 29 30
```

MAY
```
 S  M  T  W  T  F  S
             1  2
 3  4  5  6  7  8  9
10 11 12 13 14 15 16
17 18 19 20 21 22 23
24/31 25 26 27 28 29 30
```

JUNE
```
 S  M  T  W  T  F  S
    1  2  3  4  5  6
 7  8  9 10 11 12 13
14 15 16 17 18 19 20
21 22 23 24 25 26 27
28 29 30
```

JULY
```
 S  M  T  W  T  F  S
          1  2  3  4
 5  6  7  8  9 10 11
12 13 14 15 16 17 18
19 20 21 22 23 24 25
26 27 28 29 30 31
```

AUGUST
```
 S  M  T  W  T  F  S
                   1
 2  3  4  5  6  7  8
 9 10 11 12 13 14 15
16 17 18 19 20 21 22
23/30 24/31 25 26 27 28 29
```

SEPTEMBER
```
 S  M  T  W  T  F  S
       1  2  3  4  5
 6  7  8  9 10 11 12
13 14 15 16 17 18 19
20 21 22 23 24 25 26
27 28 29 30
```

OCTOBER
```
 S  M  T  W  T  F  S
             1  2  3
 4  5  6  7  8  9 10
11 12 13 14 15 16 17
18 19 20 21 22 23 24
25 26 27 28 29 30 31
```

NOVEMBER
```
 S  M  T  W  T  F  S
 1  2  3  4  5  6  7
 8  9 10 11 12 13 14
15 16 17 18 19 20 21
22 23 24 25 26 27 28
29 30
```

DECEMBER
```
 S  M  T  W  T  F  S
       1  2  3  4  5
 6  7  8  9 10 11 12
13 14 15 16 17 18 19
20 21 22 23 24 25 26
27 28 29 30 31
```

ol, coffee, and cola.

es saliva, which neutralizes acid. of sugarless gum.

the LES, stimulates stomach acid a.

ut three hours after eating before e to decrease and your stomach

Use gravity to keep stomach acid

increase acid production, and stom- overflow into your esophagus.

▸ **Wear loose clothing.** Don't wear tight-fitting clothes or belts.

- ▶ **Slim down.** If you are overweight, the extra weight squeezes your belly and forces the acidic digestive juices back up into your esophagus.

- ▶ **Reduce stress in your life.** Yoga, tai chi, and aromatherapy are some tried and true stress-relieving techniques.

Antacids and acid-suppressing drugs have their place, too. Over-the-counter remedies, such as Tums and Mylanta, neutralize acid already in your stomach. These drugs are fine for treating occasional bouts of heartburn, but experts say don't rely on them to treat chronic heartburn. Taking antacids regularly may result in rebound heartburn, where your body produces more acid to counteract the antacid.

If you suffer from heartburn more than twice a week, see your doctor about medications that can better manage your reflux. Please see *Antacids* in Chapter 6 for more information.

Chest pain

Doctors describe chest pain as mild to severe discomfort in the rib area, often under the breastbone.

Common causes. Heart conditions often trigger chest pain. It's a classic warning sign of a heart attack and heart disease. But this discomfort can have digestive and even musculoskeletal causes, too. Ulcers may radiate pain into the rib area, while acid reflux, gastroesophageal reflux disease (GERD), and esophagitis — inflammation of the esophagus — may create a burning sensation behind the breastbone. Fibromyalgia, as well as osteoarthritis and rheumatoid arthritis, can also lead to chest pain. So can anxiety disorders and panic attacks.

When to seek help. It's hard to tell the difference between chest pain linked to digestive problems and the kind caused by heart attack or heart disease. Even doctors have trouble.

Experts say that's why you should get help immediately if you develop chest pain. It could be something as minor as heartburn, but it could also be the beginnings of a heart attack. Don't take chances because the risk is too great.

Self-care. Your doctor will give you self-care advice once she knows the cause. Take chest pain seriously and seek medical care rather than trying to treat it yourself.

Nausea

Everyone feels nauseous at some point, whether from motion sickness, food poisoning, or stomach flu. It's never pleasant. You feel queasy, as if you might throw up. You may suddenly feel weak, start sweating, get the chills, turn pale, and even have a fever. Sometimes your stomach further revolts, leading to diarrhea, cramps, bloating, and vomiting.

Common causes. Nausea is a common symptom of many conditions, including these:

▶ viral infection or stomach flu

▶ food poisoning

▶ motion sickness, seasickness, or vertigo

▶ overeating

▶ blocked intestine

▶ migraine headache

▶ unsettling smells, thoughts, or sights, such as seeing someone else vomit

▶ emotional stress or fear

▶ concussion or brain injury

▶ exposure to chemical toxins

Several medicines, such as antibiotics, count nausea among their side effects. The same is true of some supplements, including herbs. Read labels carefully, and ask your doctor about the potential side effects of any medication or supplement you are taking.

When to seek help. Most often, nausea is not serious, but occasionally it stems from more serious problems, like ulcers, gallstones, pancreatitis, liver disease, kidney disease, heatstroke, heart attack, and brain tumor. You may also experience it with infections, like appendicitis, encephalitis, or meningitis, and some forms of cancer.

Watch for warning signs of a more serious problem, such as appendicitis, and call your doctor immediately or go to the emergency room of the nearest hospital if you develop any of these symptoms along with nausea.

- vomit that's bloody or looks like coffee grounds
- fever of 101 degrees Fahrenheit or higher
- diarrhea
- rapid breathing or pulse
- severe abdominal pain
- confusion
- agonizing headache
- stiff neck
- severe fatigue

Self-care. Although nausea may cause severe discomfort, in many cases, you can treat or prevent it with tried-and-true home remedies.

- *Eat smaller, more frequent meals* instead of three big meals a day. Eat and drink slowly.
- *Drink liquids between meals* instead of with them to avoid overly distending your stomach.
- *Try not to mix* hot and cold foods.

▸ *Stay away from fried,* greasy, or sweet foods that may upset your tummy.

▸ *Stick to cold or room-temperature foods* if the smell of hot or warm foods upsets your stomach.

▸ *Avoid activity after you eat.* Rest instead. Keep your head elevated 12 inches above your feet. Also, do not brush your teeth immediately after eating.

▸ *Try over-the-counter bismuth solutions*, like Pepto-Bismol to relieve simple nausea.

Motion sickness is even easier to thwart. Follow these simple guidelines for a smooth ride.

▸ *Face front while traveling,* and resist looking out the side windows of a moving vehicle.

▸ *Avoid strong odors,* like cologne or smoke, and get some fresh air.

▸ *Eat lightly about three hours before traveling.* Stay away from dairy products and foods high in protein, salt, or calories. Don't smoke or drink before leaving on a trip.

▸ *Try acupressure.* Evidence suggests wristbands specially designed to prevent motion sickness may actually work.

▸ *Take ginger to settle your upset stomach.* It comes in several forms, including powder, capsules, candied, crystallized, or tea. Turmeric, a spice found in curry dishes, may also help.

▸ *Look for antihistamines,* such as dimenhydrinate (Dramamine) or meclizine (Bonine or Dramamine II) at your favorite drugstore. Although these antihistamines can all cause drowsiness, meclizine is preferred because it causes less drowsiness.

▸ *Consider wearing a skin patch,* like scopolamine (Transderm Scop). Recent research suggests that patches, which provide a steady stream of medicine, may be more effective than oral medication.

Bloating

Bloating is that uncomfortable feeling of stretching, distention, and trapped gas you feel after eating a large meal or drinking a carbonated beverage.

Common causes. Intestinal gas comes from two places — air you swallow and gas created by bacteria living in your large intestine as they digest food.

But experts say, surprisingly, that people who complain of bloating don't swallow more air or produce more gas than other people. Instead, the gas moves more slowly through their digestive tract. Sometimes, it even moves backward, returning to the stomach. Gas passes more slowly out of the body, so it has time to accumulate, stretching the bowels and making life very uncomfortable.

Some people, like those with IBS, are also more sensitive to gas. They feel the stretching in their bowels more acutely than other people, so the bloating is more bothersome. Often when your stomach is upset, your insides are more sensitive than usual, and you feel bloated.

Weak abdominal muscles may also play a role. Many people say their bloating begins during the day and becomes worse right after dinner. Experts think this pattern points to weak abdominal muscles, especially in women who have had one or more children.

When to seek help. It's not usually a serious problem, but sometimes bloating could be a warning sign of other hidden health problems, like irritable bowel syndrome, Crohn's disease, colon cancer, or some hernias. Trapped gas can also mimic serious conditions, like heart disease.

See your doctor if:

▶ the location of your abdominal pain changes.

▶ the pain suddenly becomes much worse or strikes more often.

▶ you are over 40 years old and develop new symptoms along with bloating.

Self-care. Don't put up with annoying bloating. You can battle it with a few feel-good tips.

▶ *Start banishing high-fat foods* from your table, like red meats, cream, butter, nuts, and seeds. You digest them slowly, and this can make you feel painfully bloated.

▶ *Back off on whipped and fizzy foods,* like soufflés, milkshakes, whipped cream, and carbonated drinks and see if you notice an improvement.

▶ *Sprinkle a half-tablespoon of the spice turmeric,* a key ingredient of curry dishes, on food to neutralize that bloated and sick feeling. But beware of turmeric if you have gallbladder problems as it could aggravate them.

▶ *Avoid overeating at one big meal.* Instead, eat several smaller meals throughout the day.

▶ *Take a leisurely walk after meals.* Don't lie down or sit slouched over after eating.

▶ *See if your bloating feels better when you lie down* and worsens when you stand up. If so, weak abdominal muscles may be to blame. Try strengthening and tightening your midsection with sit-ups and other exercises.

▶ *Get some exercise.* Sometimes exercise will help move gas along through your digestive system.

▶ *Try gas-relieving medicine,* like simethicone, available in many over-the-counter antacids. Just be aware that not everyone gets gas relief from this ingredient.

Belching

When you eat, you swallow air along with your food. When you eat or drink too fast, or when you drink something fizzy, you swallow even more air. Belching, or burping, is nothing more than the escape of that air through your mouth.

Common causes. All burps come from swallowed air. According to the American College of Gastroenterology, you could be belching excessively if you:

▸ wear poorly fitting dentures.

▸ chew gum or suck on hard candies.

▸ swallow too much as a nervous habit or due to postnasal drip.

▸ don't thoroughly chew your food.

▸ smoke.

When to seek help. Burping is usually nothing to fret over, but chronic, repetitive burping may indicate a peptic ulcer, GERD (gastroesophageal reflux disease), or other upper gastrointestinal disorder.

Self-care. Drink slowly, without gulping air, to reduce belching. And stop drinking out of small-mouthed bottles or through a straw. This will cut down on how much air makes it to your stomach. Don't rush through your meal. Eat slowly and chew carefully and you'll swallow less air.

Gas

Gas is usually a reminder that your gastrointestinal, or GI, tract is alive and well. When it escapes at the entrance, it presents itself as burping. When it's stuck in the middle, it's bloating. When it escapes through the exit, it's called "breaking wind."

Common causes. Passing gas has plenty of nicknames, but it's both correct and polite to speak of it as flatulence — the passing of flatus. These vapors in your digestive tract come from two places — swallowed air and the digestion of certain foods in your large intestine.

Some foods produce more gas than others. These foods aren't completely processed until they reach your colon where bacteria finish breaking them down, producing gas in the process.

Most flatus is odorless, especially gas produced in the colon by beneficial bacteria acting on soluble fiber. But sometimes these bacteria release sulfur-containing gases as they digest food, mainly food like eggs that contain sulfur. This can cause embarrassing odors.

When to seek help. On its own, gas is nothing much to worry about. The American College of Gastroenterology says it's normal to pass flatus up to 20 times a day.

In rare cases, excessive gas points to food intolerances, such as lactose intolerance or celiac disease, where your body cannot digest the gluten in grains. Speak with your doctor if you're concerned about the amount of gas you pass, or if you develop excessive gas along with any of these symptoms.

- abdominal pain
- heartburn
- vomiting
- diarrhea or constipation
- weight loss
- gastrointestinal bleeding

Your doctor may run tests to rule out other conditions and can prescribe a special, low-gas diet if necessary.

Self-care. When it comes to gas and foods, you'll find both good news and bad. The bad news is you can't cut out all gas-producing foods without seriously endangering your health. Any food that contains sugar, starch, or soluble fiber can potentially cause gas.

The good news is foods that give one person gas may not bother another. Keep track of what you eat in a daily food diary, and make note of any digestive problems you develop, like gas. This will help you pin-point which foods give you that bloated, about-to-explode feeling.

Here are some of the main culprits, along with ideas to reduce the unpleasant effects.

Defuse the foods that "explode" in your bowel

Problem food	Solution
Cabbage	Try seasoning cooked cabbage with caraway seeds to cut down on gas.
Beans	Change the water you cook the beans in several times, or add a few drops of Beano, an anti-gas food enzyme, to them after cooking.
Cucumbers	Choose the "burpless," or seedless, variety, since the seeds are the main source of gas.
Turnips	Skip the turnip and eat the greens. They're full of gut-friendly fiber plus anti-aging antioxidants.
Garlic	Chew a sprig of parsley after a garlic-rich meal to freshen your breath and diffuse gas.
Onions	Flavor foods with spices and herbs that are gentler on your digestive tract.
Carbonated drinks	Pour soda into a glass first to cut down on fizz or, better yet, trade it in for tea or water.
Nuts	The high-fat content of nuts can spell gassy trouble, especially if you suffer with IBS. Eat them sparingly if they upset your stomach.

Some natural sugars and artificial sweeteners can give you gas, too.

▸ raffinose – a complex sugar found in beans, cabbage, brussels sprouts, broccoli, and asparagus

▸ sucrose – the common chemical name for table sugar

▸ sorbitol and mannitol – found in many new low-sugar products

▸ fructose – a fruit sugar in pears, honey, onions, artichokes, and wheat

More tips to deflate that about-to-explode feeling:

▸ **Give digestive aids a try.** They may allow you to eat foods that normally give you gas. Examples include Beano for beans and Lactaid, Lactrase, and Dairy Ease for dairy products.

▸ **Try anise, fennel, peppermint, caraway, or chamomile.** The oils or seeds from some herbs can halt gas — even better than some store-bought solutions.

▸ **Deflate stomach gas with antacids,** but they won't do much for intestinal gas.

▸ **Try taking activated charcoal caplets.** Some health experts think they can help.

▸ **Ease the cramps that often come with gas** by taking anti-spasmodic drugs, but talk with your doctor about potential side effects.

▸ **Avoid using cold medications for long periods** of time and you may see your gas symptoms disappear, according to the American College of Gastroenterology.

▸ **Banish the embarrassing odor of intestinal gas** with Devrom, an over-the-counter tablet containing bismuth subgallate. Bismuth kills anaerobic bacteria that produce foul-smelling gas in the first place.

Vomiting

Several things happen when your body sends your brain a signal to vomit. First, the esophageal sphincter that separates your stomach and esophagus relaxes. Then the abdominal muscles and diaphragm contract, and your windpipe closes. Last, the muscles wrapped around your stomach squeeze violently, pushing your stomach's contents up your esophagus and out your mouth.

Common causes. Lots of conditions can trigger vomiting, everything from stress and anxiety to inner ear problems. Here are some of the other common culprits.

- viral or bacterial infections
- migraine headache
- motion sickness
- food poisoning
- medication
- obstruction in the intestine, caused by ulcers, cancer, or inflammatory bowel disease, such as Crohn's
- irritation or inflammation of the stomach, small intestine, or gallbladder

You can sometimes tell what's causing you to vomit by the timing. Chronic vomiting during or right after a meal could indicate a peptic ulcer. Ingesting a toxic substance tends to trigger vomiting within eight hours. Viral or bacterial infections may take longer to make you ill.

When to seek help. Generally, if the vomiting is short-lived, and if you know the likely cause — like carsickness, a virus, or spoiled food — you can simply wait for it to pass. But watch closely for other symptoms. See a doctor right away if you:

- develop a fever of 101 degrees Fahrenheit or higher.
- have severe abdominal pain.

- get diarrhea.

- start sweating heavily.

- have vomit that's bloody or looks like coffee grounds.

- become confused or severely fatigued.

- develop an agonizing headache or a stiff neck.

- smell a slight odor of feces in your vomit.

- experience explosive, projectile vomiting.

Self-care. Vomiting takes a lot out of you, energy as well as nutrients. Rest, try to stay hydrated, and begin eating easy-to-digest foods once your stomach calms down.

- *Be sure to get plenty of liquids.* At first, stick to clear, ice-cold drinks, such as water or clear sodas. Drinks containing sugar calm the stomach better than other liquids. Stay away from acidic juices, like orange or grapefruit.

- *Drink clear liquids every half hour* if you also have diarrhea. You can slowly try caffeine-free sodas, clear broth, and weak tea. Peppermint and chamomile tea, in particular, can help soothe your stomach.

- *Gradually add gentle foods.* Try the BRAT diet of bananas, rice, applesauce, and toast to ease back into solid foods. Bland foods, like broth, gelatin, saltine crackers, or plain bread, also work well.

- *Take care of yourself if you get the stomach flu.* Rest in bed and drink plenty of liquids once you can keep them down. Water and rehydrating drinks, like Gatorade, are best. Dehydration is the main concern with prolonged vomiting.

Difficulty swallowing

It's easy to take something as simple as swallowing for granted. Dysphagia, the inability to swallow or difficulty in swallowing, could change that. Simply eating enough to stay healthy could become a major challenge.

Ever get choked up over a sad movie or during an argument? Strong emotions can cause the muscles in your throat to tense up, giving you the feeling of having a "lump in your throat" when none is there. That lump, called globus sensation, comes from tightened muscles around your pharynx — the small opening at the base of your throat.

Anxiety, grief, anger, pride, happiness, and other emotions tend to create this sensation, but so can antihistamines and drugs for high blood pressure and depression. Having a cold, cough, dry throat, acid reflux, hiatal hernia, swallowing frequently, or being overweight may also play a role. This feeling should go away in a couple of days, once the muscles have loosened. If it doesn't, see your doctor.

Common causes. Swallowing is the first part of digestion and involves three stages. First, food is chewed and mixed with saliva to make it the right size and consistency to go down your throat. Next, your tongue pushes the food back. This triggers the swallowing reflex. At this point, your voice box closes and breathing stops to keep food out of your windpipe. Finally, the food travels down your esophagus to your stomach.

Dysphagia can interfere at any point in this process. Causes of swallowing problems range from a small esophagus and poor eating habits to acid reflux and disorders like stroke, Parkinson's disease, and Lou Gehrig's disease. But some problems are hard to explain — like someone who can swallow food but not pills.

Symptoms like these will tell you whether you may be suffering from dysphagia:

▸ choking, coughing, or feeling like food is sticking when you try to swallow

▸ chest pain when you eat

▸ coughing or spitting up food long after you've eaten

When to seek help. Occasional trouble swallowing shouldn't worry you. First, try eating slower and chewing your food thoroughly. See your doctor if your swallowing problem lasts more than a few days or you notice blood in your stool or vomit.

Treatment for dysphagia depends on where your swallowing mechanism has broken down. If trouble starts in your mouth and upper throat, a speech specialist may train you to swallow correctly.

Your doctor may prescribe medicine to help your throat muscles relax, such as nitroglycerin or calcium channel blockers. She may also tell you to avoid certain drugs that can irritate your esophagus, like aspirin, antihistamines, ACE inhibitors, and others. More serious esophageal problems may need medical therapy or surgery.

Self-care. Check out these sensible ways to make swallowing easier.

- ▶ *Sip water* with meals.

- ▶ *Eat slowly,* take small bites, and — most important — chew thoroughly.

- ▶ *Sit upright* while you eat.

- ▶ *Avoid cold* foods.

- ▶ *Take medications with water,* while sitting up, and well before bedtime.

- ▶ *Treat acid* reflux.

- ▶ *Be sure your dentures* are secure.

For more information

Contact these organizations for more information about dysphagia and a list of support groups.

International Foundation for Functional Gastrointestinal Disorders Inc.
P.O. Box 170864
Milwaukee, WI 53217
888–964–2001 or
414–964–1799
www.iffgd.org

American Speech-Language-Hearing Association
10801 Rockville Pike
Rockville, MD 20852
800-638-8255
www.asha.org/public/speech

▶ *Find qualified help* from a throat specialist, neurologist, speech-language pathologist, or physical therapist.

Dysphagia can put you at risk for malnutrition and dehydration. The challenge is to eat enough nutritious food to stay healthy.

Thanks to blenders, you can make almost anything in a balanced, nutritious diet easy to swallow. Use trial and error to find a consistency that suits you.

Abdominal pain

It comes in many shapes and sizes — sometimes as dull, cramping pain low in your gut; sharp, stabbing pains in your midsection; or a burning sensation in your stomach.

Common causes. Almost any digestive problem and many nondigestive conditions can trigger this discomfort. Digestive diseases sometimes cause referred pain, or pain in another part of your body far away from the source of the problem.

For instance, a gallbladder attack may cause pain in your shoulder blade. And likewise, some nondigestive problems can cause abdominal pain, such as a heart attack. The chart on the following page shows the types of pain certain conditions tend to cause.

For more information about specific conditions that commonly cause abdominal pain, please see Chapter 3.

When to seek help. Pain that lasts only a few moments then goes away isn't cause for alarm. On the other hand, you should definitely see your doctor if the pain lasts longer than several hours, or if you experience any of these red-flag symptoms.

▶ fever

▶ loss of appetite or weight

Pain characteristics	Potential causes
Cramping pain in the abdomen	Excess gas; intestinal irritation from infection, inflammation, intestinal blockage, or stress
Cramping waves of pain along with loud grumbling sounds in abdomen	Blocked intestines
Steady pain, as a burn, ache, or sharp pain	Ulcers; gallstones; acid reflux; infections of any abdominal organ; blood, bile, or intestinal contents leaking into abdominal cavity
Steady pain along with a sloshing sound in stomach	Ulcer blocking end of stomach
Abdominal pain accompanied by nausea or vomiting	Blockage in stomach, intestine, or gallbladder; inflammation of pancreas
Cramping pain along with black or bloody stool	Severe internal bleeding
Pain accompanied by dark, tea-like urine and light stool	Blocked bile duct
Hunger or gnawing pain relieved by eating	Peptic ulcer
Occurs in center of upper abdomen	Problem with esophagus, stomach, duodenum, liver, pancreas, or bile ducts

Continued

Pain characteristics	Potential causes
Occurs on right side of upper abdomen	Gallbladder, inflamed liver
Radiates into back	Ulcer, irritation of pancreas
Localized pain around navel	Problem with small intestine
Localized pain below navel to the right, left, or middle of abdomen	Problem with large intestine
Uncomfortable pressure around rectum	Condition inside pelvic area
Strikes just before mealtime	Peptic ulcer
Strikes after meals	Problem with gallbladder or pancreas, intestinal obstruction
Triggered by swallowing hot or cold foods	Esophageal problem
Relieved by pacing or rocking	Blockage in intestine or gallbladder
Relieved by lying down and drawing up legs	Appendicitis
Relieved by leaning forward or curling into a ball on one side	Inflammation of pancreas
Creates trouble swallowing food or saliva	Irritation or blockage of esophagus

- diarrhea or persistent constipation
- change in bowel habits
- blood in stool or vomit
- continual nausea or vomiting
- abdominal swelling
- severe tenderness in belly
- jaundice
- trouble swallowing
- pain that wakes you up
- steady, severe, or regularly occurring pain
- previous history of ulcers, acid reflux, gallstones, ulcerative colitis, Crohn's disease, or intestinal surgery

If your abdominal discomfort feels like general indigestion, try settling it with some of these remedies:

- bitter foods, such as watercress, endive, dandelion greens, artichokes, grated orange peel, and ginger
- chamomile tea

Self-care. Your doctor will be able to advise you on how to care for yourself once she knows the cause of your abdominal pain.

Diarrhea

The average person gets diarrhea four times a year, but just because it's a regular visitor doesn't mean you should ignore it.

Common causes. Normally, your digestive system absorbs all the fluid and nutrients it needs from what you've eaten and leaves the rest in the form of solid stool to pass out of your body. When you suffer from diarrhea, food passes too quickly through your colon, and it can't absorb fluids like it should. In some cases, the lining of your colon is inflamed or unhealthy and unable to work properly. The result is loose, watery, and more frequent stools.

Diarrhea: a symptom with many origins

Organism (Infection)	Symptoms	How you get it
Campylobacter jejuni (Campylobacteriosis)	watery or sticky diarrhea (may be bloody); abdominal pain; nausea; fever; headache; muscle pain	Bacterial food poisoning *Common sources*: improperly cooked chicken, raw milk, and untreated water
Clostridium perfringens (Perfringens food poisoning)	diarrhea; intense abdominal cramps	Bacterial food poisoning *Common sources*: raw meat, poultry, and eggs, as well as meat and gravy not properly refrigerated
E. coli 0157:H7 (Hemorrhagic colitis)	watery diarrhea that may become grossly bloody; severe abdominal cramps; sometimes vomiting and fever	Bacterial food poisoning *Common sources*: undercooked beef, unpasteurized apple juice or cider, alfalfa sprouts, and lettuce
Entamoeba histolytica (Amebiasis)	may vary from no symptoms to severe symptoms, such as diarrhea with blood and mucus	Food and water contaminated with parasite from feces *Common sources*: poor hygiene and sexual contact
Giardia lamblia (Giardiasis)	mild to severe, foul-smelling, yellow diarrhea; fatigue; abdominal pain, cramps, and bloating; no fever or blood in stool	Water contaminated with parasite from feces or transmission of the parasite from someone already contaminated
Salmonella (Salmonellosis)	"pea soup" diarrhea; nausea and vomiting; abdominal cramps; fever; headache	Bacterial food poisoning *Common sources*: raw meats, poultry, eggs, dairy products, fish, sauces, and salad dressings

Continued

Conditions	Symptoms	Common causes
Shigella (Shigellosis or bacillary dysentery)	diarrhea; blood, pus, or mucus in the stool; fever; abdominal cramps; vomiting	Bacterial food poisoning *Common sources:* salads, like potato and macaroni, dairy products, poultry, raw vegetables, contaminated water, and poor hygiene
V. cholerae (Cholera)	mild, watery diarrhea to acute diarrhea, with "rice water" stool; abdominal cramps; nausea and vomiting	Bacterial food poisoning *Common sources:* raw or improperly cooked shellfish from contaminated waters
Viruses (Viral gastroenteritis or "stomach flu")	diarrhea; nausea and vomiting; mild fever; abdominal cramps	Viral infection from one of many different viruses *Common sources:* direct contact with infected person or sharing food, drink, or utensils
Crohn's disease	urgent diarrhea; abdominal pain; fatigue; weight loss	Small intestine and colon most commonly affected *Likely causes:* genetic and environmental factors
Food allergy or intolerance	diarrhea; abdominal pain; itching; hives; dizziness, lightheadedness	Immune system reaction, often triggered by certain proteins in food *Common triggers:* Eggs, peanuts, shellfish, and tree nuts
Irritable bowel syndrome (IBS)	painful diarrhea (sometimes mucus in stool); cramping; bloating; gas; constipation	Disorder in which nerves and muscles of the bowel are extra sensitive *Common triggers:* Stress, food, exercise, and hormones
Ulcerative colitis	urgent and bloody diarrhea; abdominal pain; fatigue	Inflammation of the colon, or large intestine *Likely causes:* genetic and environmental factors

There are technically two types of diarrhea, acute and chronic. Acute diarrhea lasts a short period of time and has a temporary cause, such as:

- food poisoning
- parasites
- bacterial infections
- viral infections
- a reaction to artificial sweeteners
- a side effect of some drugs, such as antibiotics

Chronic diarrhea stays around much longer because it's caused by a problem in your digestive system that won't go away on its own, such as:

- gastroenteritis
- inflammatory bowel disease
- irritable bowel syndrome
- diverticular disease
- food intolerance
- intestinal blockage
- malabsorption
- fecal impaction

When to seek help. Run-of-the-mill diarrhea usually lasts one or two days with bowel movements more than three times a day. You might also experience cramping, bloating, fever, or nausea. This kind of diarrhea will often go away on its own. See a doctor if:

- you still have diarrhea after three days. She can perform tests to determine what's making you ill.
- you develop bad stomach pain, a high fever, dehydration, or blood in your stool along with diarrhea.

Acute diarrhea might only require medication, while chronic diarrhea means involving your doctor and perhaps changing your lifestyle.

Self-care. Your doctor will give you a specific eating plan if a more serious condition is causing your diarrhea. Otherwise, your goal is to help your body get through this short-term ordeal.

▶ *Stay away from milk* and greasy or high-fiber foods. These will only aggravate your system.

▶ *Skip food and candy with artificial sweeteners,* since they can cause diarrhea.

▶ *Begin eating soft, carbohydrate-rich foods,* like potatoes, oatmeal, and noodles, when you start to feel better. Some doctors recommend the easy-to-remember BRAT diet — Bananas, Rice, Applesauce, and Toast.

▶ *Keep your body hydrated.* Signs of dangerous dehydration include thirst, fatigue, dry skin, dark urine, feeling lightheaded, and not needing to urinate as much as usual. Severe dehydration can be fatal. Call your doctor or go immediately to an emergency room if you experience dehydration associated with severe diarrhea.

▶ *Replenish the fluids and electrolytes* — potassium and sodium — your body needs to function by adding broth, soup, soft fruit, fruit juice, clear soda, and gelatin to your diet. To make a rehydration drink at home, add a half teaspoon of salt and eight teaspoons of sugar to one liter (a little more than a quart) of water. You can also add a half cup of fruit juice or a mashed, ripe banana to the mixture for extra potassium.

If you're constantly having bouts of diarrhea, help your doctor determine the cause, and you'll be that much closer to a solution. Start with a food diary and write down everything you eat. Then write down your bathroom habits. You may see a connection between the diarrhea and certain foods. This can be especially helpful in ferreting out conditions like lactose intolerance.

▶ *Avoid alcohol and caffeine* while you have diarrhea. These will only dehydrate you more.

▶ *Over-the-counter* products containing loperamide or bismuth subsalicylate — like Imodium, Pepto Bismol, and Kaopectate — can make life a little easier when you're suffering from diarrhea. But remember, they will only reduce the symptoms, not treat the underlying problem.

▶ *Never take anti-diarrhea* products when a parasite or bacterial infection is the cause of your trouble. Your body needs to flush the intruder out of your system. Stopping the diarrhea will make the situation worse. However, there is a very important exception to this advice. If diarrhea is severe, dehydration can be fatal. In this case, stopping severe diarrhea is the first priority.

Simple exercise keeps you in control

Bowel incontinence is an inconvenience you can live without. About 10 percent of Americans lose at least some control over their bowel movements. But a simple exercise could prevent the embarrassment of both bowel and urinary incontinence.

Pelvic floor, or Kegel, exercises strengthen the bladder and bowel in addition to giving you peace of mind. And they are so discreet, you can do them anywhere.

You will need to squeeze two groups of muscles — the ones around your anus, as if you are trying to keep from passing gas, and the muscles under your bladder, as if you are trying to stop the flow of urine. Tighten both sets of muscles, count to four, and release. It's that simple.

Aim to do this at least 30 times, 3 times a day for long-term results. Start by exercising while lying down. As you get stronger, do the Kegels while sitting or standing. Continue to exercise in all three positions daily — lying, sitting, and standing — to better strengthen your muscles.

You can protect yourself from getting diarrhea in the first place by practicing a few smart habits.

- ▶ **Wash your hands often** to protect yourself from viral diarrhea, which spreads easily from person to person.

- ▶ **Cut down on diarrhea caused by contaminated food** by practicing safe cooking and food storage.

- ▶ **Be aware of the medications you take.** Some can trigger diarrhea as a side effect. A French medical study suggests NSAIDs (non-steroidal anti-inflammatory drugs), such as aspirin and ibuprofen, increase the risk of acute diarrhea. Antacids, antibiotics, and certain heart medicines can also cause diarrhea.

Constipation

Some health professionals say you don't need to have a bowel movement every day. Many others think infrequent bowel movements are not normal for people who have adequate fiber in their diet.

Doctors write more than 1 million prescriptions a year to treat constipation. It's easier than you think to relieve constipation naturally without drugs. But take steps if you have two or more of these symptoms.

- ▶ You have fewer than three bowel movements a week.

- ▶ About a quarter of your bowel movements require straining.

- ▶ You feel like you still need to go after at least a quarter of your bowel movements.

- ▶ A quarter of your bowel movements produce hard, pellet-like stools.

If you're constipated, you may also experience bloating, gas, and that too-full feeling.

Common causes. Normally, muscles in your colon wall move waste along at the right speed. This gives your colon time to pull water from the waste. But sometimes things don't move along quickly enough and too much water is removed. You're left with dry, hard stool, and constipation sets in.

Some health experts think aging causes this colon slowdown, but most experts say the blame belongs elsewhere. You might find yourself constipated — at any age — if you:

▸ eat less fiber than your body needs. Low-fiber convenience foods tempt all ages, but especially single, older adults who have lost interest in eating.

▸ don't get enough exercise. People of all ages have this problem, but certain health conditions or prescribed bed rest are more likely to prevent older adults from exercising.

▸ take certain medications, including sedatives, diuretics, antidepressants, aluminum or calcium antacids, iron or calcium supplements, cough syrup with codeine, and antihistamines.

▸ don't drink enough fluids. As you age, your body loses its ability to make you feel thirsty. People may even avoid drinking water because they have trouble swallowing, suffer from incontinence, or find it difficult to get up to use the bathroom.

▸ suffer from colon conditions, like inflammatory bowel disease or irritable bowel syndrome.

▸ have diabetes, low thyroid activity, depression, Parkinson's disease, heart disease, and several other health conditions.

▸ haven't learned to manage your stress.

When to seek help. First, try fiber, exercise, and fluids. If your constipation hasn't improved after a week, see your doctor. Constipation can be a symptom of many serious conditions, including diverticular disease, diabetes, and slowed thyroid activity. Make an immediate appointment if you:

▸ suddenly become constipated for no apparent reason.

▶ have mysterious weight loss.

▶ notice unexplained bleeding from your rectum.

▶ develop severe abdominal pain.

Self-care. Lack of daily bowel movements doesn't necessarily mean you're constipated, but this is an indication that you aren't getting enough fiber in your diet. Try these seven ways to beat constipation, without medicine or a doctor's visit.

▶ *Gradually add fiber* to your diet until you're getting at least the minimum recommended daily amount of 21 grams for women and 30 grams for men. If you're not meeting this goal, try eating more whole grains, fruits, beans, and vegetables.

▶ *Back off on meat* and dairy products. Foods that are high in fat and low in fiber may contribute to constipation.

▶ *Eat slowly* and chew your food well.

▶ *Get regular with exercise.* A mild workout stimulates your bowels. In fact, you can ease constipation with your feet. Simply walking may work better than any pill, laxative, or medicine.

▶ *Visit the bathroom* at the same time each day. Establishing a pattern for your bowels — perhaps in the morning after breakfast — can help you go like clockwork to avoid constipation and stay on track.

Some experts say if you overuse laxatives you could become dependent on them, developing chronic constipation and weak intestines. Others disagree.

Bulk-forming laxatives, including psyllium (Metamucil), methylcellulose (Citrucel), calcium polycarbophil (Fibercon), and bran — are the safest kinds, although they may keep your body from absorbing 100 percent of certain medicines.

Most laxatives are short-term treatments for occasional constipation. Discuss the options with your doctor if you need long-term help staying regular.

However, don't force the issue by rushing or straining. And if you need to go at another time, answer nature's call without trying to wait.

▶ *Massage your abdominal area* in a clockwise motion. Some natural healers believe this helps relieve constipation. Therapeutic massage also shows promise as a remedy for constipation, which can be triggered or worsened by stress.

▶ *Try simple relaxation techniques,* like sitting quietly for 15 to 20 minutes each day, focusing on deep, even breathing.

To beat constipation naturally remember the two F's — fiber and fluids. The fiber in whole grains, fruits, vegetables, and beans acts as a natural laxative, making your stool soft enough to pass quickly and smoothly through your system.

When you add more fiber to your diet and drink lots of water, constipation may not be the only thing that gets better. Sometimes treating constipation helps ease heartburn, as well.

But without water or other liquids, all that fiber could cause an intestinal blockage. Liquids will keep food moving through your digestive tract and help the fiber soften your stool for easy elimination. Drink at least six to eight glasses of liquids every day.

Bleeding

Bleeding from your digestive tract can come out through your mouth or anus. Passing blood is always alarming and sometimes, but not always, serious.

Common causes. A minor problem, like hemorrhoids, could be to blame, or more serious conditions, like inflammatory bowel disease, ulcer, diverticulosis, or cancer may be culprits. Or you may have esophagitis, gastritis, a large hiatal hernia, an anal fissure, or a tear in your esophagus. Aspirin and other nonsteroidal anti-inflammatory drugs can also lead to bleeding in your digestive tract.

The color of the blood and where it comes out give doctors clues about the cause.

> Blood in the stool can show up either bright red or black. But sometimes black stools are caused by the bismuth in medicines, such as Pepto-Bismol. See your doctor if you have any doubts.

▸ Vomited blood, whether bright red or the color of coffee grounds, usually points to a problem in your upper digestive tract.

▸ Dark, tar-like stools generally indicate bleeding in your upper digestive tract from your esophagus, stomach, or small intestine. For instance, it may come from a peptic ulcer.

▸ Bright red blood in your stool suggests a source in your lower intestinal tract, like your large intestine or rectum, perhaps from diverticulosis or hemorrhoids.

When to seek help. See your doctor as soon as you notice evidence of blood in your stool, saliva, or vomit. It may turn out to be a minor problem, but you are better safe than sorry.

Self-care. Do not attempt to treat yourself for internal bleeding. See your doctor immediately and let her determine the cause. Together you can decide the best course of treatment.

Weight loss

Everyone gains or loses a few pounds over time, but sudden, unexplainable weight loss may point to a serious digestive disorder.

Common causes. Many things can trigger weight loss. Here are a few potential causes.

- difficulty swallowing (dysphagia)

- ulcers with abdominal pain

- inflammatory bowel disease, including Crohn's disease and ulcerative colitis, especially if you develop diarrhea or bloody stools

- liver disease or diseases of the pancreas, including pancreatitis

- digestive cancer

- malabsorption disorder, such as Celiac disease

- skipping meals or other changes in diet

- increases in activity, such as starting a new exercise program or job

- certain herbs and medications, including some antidepressants and stimulants

- changes in mood, like depression, anxiety, or stress

When to seek help. Keep track of your weight. Small fluctuations are normal, but see your doctor if you have unintentionally lost 5 percent of your body weight in a few weeks or 10 percent of your body weight in the last six months. He can determine the cause, give you a healthy weight-gain meal plan, and monitor future changes.

Self-care. Make sure you eat at least three-balanced meals every day. For snacks or missed meals, consider nutritional supplement drinks. See your doctor if you have followed a balanced meal plan for two weeks and still have not stopped losing weight, or if you suspect a medication or health problem is causing your weight loss.

CHAPTER 3

Digestive problems

YOUR DIGESTIVE SYSTEM IS LIKE THE ENGINE IN A CAR. It has lots of delicate parts, and what you put in it has a big effect on how well it runs. Occasionally something is bound to stop working. This chapter is your owner's manual. You will learn about common digestive ailments, including specific symptoms, how to lower your risk, successful medical therapies, and home remedies that really work.

Esophageal diverticula
Secret cause of bad breath

Esophageal diverticula are pouches that form along your esophagus, the tube connecting your mouth to your stomach. When you swallow, food should move smoothly down this passageway. But when you have esophageal diverticula, food gets trapped in these pouches. This can affect your ability to swallow, and it may be the secret cause of your bad breath.

What causes esophageal diverticula?

The pouches develop when something else is wrong with your esophagus, such as esophageal muscle spasms, weak muscles, narrowed spots, or problems with the lower esophageal sphincter.

These breakdowns increase the pressure inside your esophagus when you swallow, so food moving down pushes harder against the walls. Weak spots along the esophagus eventually start to give and stretch out when you swallow. At first, the wall may bulge just a little, but over time, a permanent pouch may form.

Experts recognize three types of esophageal diverticulum, based on where the pouch forms along the esophagus.

- Zenker's, or pulsion, diverticula form high up, in the pharynx (throat).
- Mid-esophageal, or traction, diverticula form midway down the esophagus.
- Epiphrenic diverticula form farther down the esophagus, just above the stomach.

When to seek help

Swallowing is a complex process, and many things can go wrong. These conditions offer a few examples. See your doctor if you notice any of the associated symptoms. She may be able to suggest lifestyle changes and prescribe medicine to bring you relief. In a few extreme cases, surgery may be necessary.

▶ In erosive esophagitis, areas of the esophageal lining become inflamed and wear away, resulting in pain and difficulty swallowing. Long-term acid reflux can cause this erosion. So can pills, such as aspirin, and other NSAIDs if they get stuck in your esophagus and dissolve, eating away the lining.

▶ Mallory-Weiss syndrome occurs when strong or prolonged vomiting tears the lining of your esophagus, which leads to esophageal bleeding. You may vomit the blood or pass it with stool in a few hours to a few days.

▶ In achalasia, the ring of muscles known as the lower esophageal sphincter at the base of your esophagus will not relax to let food into your stomach. You may regurgitate food, lose weight, or have chest pain, difficulty belching, or trouble swallowing liquids and solids, which worsens over time.

▶ Diffuse esophageal spasms are strong, prolonged contractions of the muscles lining the esophagus. These spasms may give you occasional trouble swallowing both liquids and solid food, as well as pain behind the breastbone.

▶ Stricture is a narrowing of the esophagus due to chronic inflammation and scar tissue caused by GERD (gastroesophageal reflux disease). People with this condition have difficulty swallowing food, which gets worse over time

Common symptoms and early warning signs

Small esophageal diverticula may produce no symptoms, but large ones can. Sometimes the symptoms are subtle — bad breath, hoarseness, chronic coughing, or a bad taste in your mouth. Other signs are more bothersome.

> ▶ difficulty swallowing (dysphagia)

> ▶ heartburn

> ▶ coughing up or regurgitating food, even hours after eating it, especially when bending over or lying down

> ▶ pneumonia

Are you at risk?

Men are three times more likely than women to develop esophageal diverticula. Middle-age men tend to develop epiphrenic diverticula, while older men over the age of 60 tend to get Zenker's. Having another esophageal disorder, such as muscle spasms, increases your chance of developing esophageal diverticula.

Medical procedure your doctor may order

Health professionals use this simple test to determine if you have esophageal diverticula.

> **Barium swallow.** After you swallow barium, a liquid contrast dye, a special X-ray machine makes moving X-rays that can show the out-pouchings of esophageal diverticula.

For more details about medical tests, see Chapter 7.

Nutritional defense against esophageal diverticula

Eating certain foods can't cure esophageal diverticula, but what and how you eat can significantly improve them.

▸ *Stick to a bland diet* whenever possible.

▸ *Eat smaller meals* throughout the day instead of two or three large ones.

▸ *Chew thoroughly* so food passes more smoothly down your esophagus.

▸ *Drink water after eating* to help wash food out of the pouch.

▸ *Puree foods* in a blender or food processor if you have trouble swallowing them.

Additional steps to take

A few simple precautions can ease the discomfort of esophageal diverticula.

▸ *Keep your head raised* while eating to help food move down your esophagus.

▸ *Stay upright* for about two hours after eating.

▸ *Control chronic coughing* with throat lozenges or other home remedies.

▸ *Avoid wearing* tight clothing.

▸ *Empty any noticeable pouches* in your neck by gently massaging them.

Medical treatment options

In most cases, making food and lifestyle changes can help you manage esophageal diverticula. Your doctor may suggest medicines to treat side effects, such as acid reflux and bad breath. In rare cases, the condition may require surgery.

▸ Antacids may dampen heartburn associated with esophageal diverticula.

▸ An over-the-counter remedy called Devrom may halt the bad breath (halitosis) resulting from decaying food trapped in esophageal diverticula. Devrom contains bismuth subgallate, a compound similar to that in Pepto Bismol, and it may kill the bacteria responsible for bad odors. Some people claim it has worked for them.

▸ Surgery to remove the pouch may be necessary in severe cases. If achalasia, or failure of the lower esophageal sphincter to relax to allow food into your stomach, caused the diverticula to develop in the first place, your doctor may also dilate the esophagus so pouches do not form again.

Talk with your doctor before taking any drugs or discontinuing any medication.

Barrett's esophagus
When heartburn spells trouble

Barrett's esophagus was named after British surgeon Norman Barrett. It affects the lining of the esophagus, the passage between your throat and stomach.

What is Barrett's esophagus?

This serious condition can develop as a complication of gastroesophageal reflux disease or GERD. As many as 12 percent of people with GERD develop Barrett's. It has also been linked with cancer of the esophagus, or esophageal cancer.

When digestive juices wash up into your esophagus, they damage the squamous epithelial cells lining the esophagus walls. Usually, your body replaces these with new squamous cells. But in the case of

Barrett's, the body replaces them with columnar epithelial cells, the kind that line your stomach.

For some reason, columnar cells in the esophagus are prone to becoming cancerous — the real danger of Barrett's. Between 5 and 10 percent of people with Barrett's develop esophageal cancer. A small risk, but the number of people with GERD and Barrett's is rising so fast that doctors fear esophageal cancer could become an epidemic. Esophageal cancer spreads quickly and widely, making it hard to cure and deadly. It kills most of its victims within one year of diagnosis.

Common symptoms and early warning signs

Barrett's does not have any symptoms of its own. Since GERD tends to cause it, watch for these signs of chronic reflux and see your doctor if you notice them alone or in combination. She can determine if you have GERD or Barrett's esophagus.

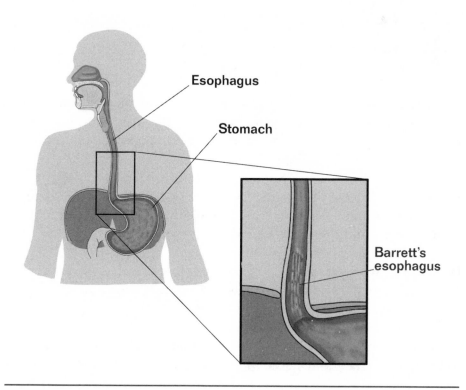

▶ heartburn two or more times a week

▶ hoarseness

▶ chronic cough

▶ wheezing similar to asthma

The following symptoms may signal something even worse, the possibility of esophageal cancer. See a doctor immediately if you experience any of these health problems.

▶ difficulty swallowing

▶ unexplained weight loss

▶ blood in vomit

▶ black or bloody stools

Are you at risk?

About 1 in 10 GERD sufferers will develop Barrett's. White, middle-age men with a long history of GERD are most at risk, but anyone can develop it, even people without GERD.

If you have Barrett's, your risk of developing esophageal cancer is about 40 times higher than someone without it. Yet, even with Barrett's, your cancer risk is small — less than one person out of 100 a year.

Some doctors blame obesity for the recent rise in GERD, and, therefore, Barrett's and esophageal cancer. Obesity raises the pressure in your stomach and intestines and, with it, your risk of acid reflux.

Diet may also play a role. The type of diet that can easily lead to obesity — too much fat and red meat and not enough fruits and vegetables — can easily cause acid reflux.

More worrisome, the acid suppressing drugs doctors commonly use to treat GERD may play a role in the rising rate of esophageal cancer.

Research shows people taking proton pump inhibitors, like Prilosec, Prevacid, or Nexium, still experience reflux. They just don't feel heartburn anymore. The kind of reflux they continue to have may do even more damage to their esophagus than before taking the drugs.

For now, experts say keep taking these medicines as your doctor ordered, but see him regularly so he can check you for signs of Barrett's esophagus and esophageal cancer.

Medical procedures your doctor may order

Barrett's esophagus can't be diagnosed based on symptoms, physical exams, or blood tests. But the following tests can help your doctor make an accurate diagnosis.

> *Upper GI endoscopy.* After throat anesthetic, you swallow a long, thin tube tipped with a tiny camera. The camera shows your esophagus on a TV monitor so your doctor can check for inflammation and erosion. If she finds trouble, she can snip a tiny amount of tissue and have it analyzed — called a biopsy — for characteristics of Barrett's cells.

> *Barium swallow.* You swallow barium, a liquid contrast dye, and X-rays are taken. The X-rays show changes in your esophagus that may be signs of Barrett's. This may be less accurate than endoscopy.

For more details about medical tests, see Chapter 7.

Nutritional defense against Barrett's esophagus

Keep a diary of the foods you eat, when you eat them, and when your heartburn occurs. Pay particular attention to these heartburn triggers.

▶ citrus fruits and juices — orange, lemon, lime, and grapefruit

▶ chocolate

▸ tomato products, including ketchup

▸ mustard, pepper, onions, garlic, and vinegar

▸ high-fat foods, especially foods high in saturated fat

Drink a thirst-quenching glass of water to help douse the flames. Remember how you get heartburn — stomach acid backs up into your esophagus and irritates it. Water helps wash the acid out.

Try drinking water about an hour before or after meals to keep your stomach from bloating. A bloated stomach is more likely to overflow, which can actually worsen reflux.

Should you be tested for Barrett's?

The burning of GERD has triggered a burning controversy. Researchers and doctors are debating whether GERD sufferers should be screened for Barrett's esophagus, which often precedes the fast-spreading esophageal cancer. Although GERD doesn't always lead to Barrett's, it has no warning signs other than frequent heartburn.

You may need to be sedated for the screening — an expensive upper GI endoscopy test to look for signs of Barrett's or cancer. Some scientists say that anyone with recurring GERD symptoms should be screened, but others suggest you should only be screened if you fit one of the two high-risk groups:

▸ you were 65 or older when you started having GERD symptoms for the first time

▸ you're a white man over 40 who has averaged two or more heartburn episodes a week for the last five years.

But keep in mind that just over 12 percent of esophageal cancer victims are women and that not everyone with GERD experiences heartburn.

Indulge in green tea often. Studies suggest people who do have less chance of getting esophageal cancer. Polyphenols, antioxidants found in tea, may prevent this type of cancer from developing. Green tea seems to pack the most polyphenols, with black and oolong teas close behind.

Additional steps to take

Controlling GERD may be the best way to prevent or limit damage from Barrett's esophagus.

- ▸ *Put a lid on heartburn.* Lose excess weight, eat smaller meals throughout the day, sit up straight when you eat, raise the head of your bed about 6 inches with blocks, steer clear of tight clothing and belts, and avoid heavy lifting and straining.

- ▸ *Ask your doctor* about the latest acid-suppressing drugs. Histamine-2 (H$_2$) blockers and proton pump inhibitors (PPIs) do a good job of lowering stomach acid levels and quelling heartburn. If your doctor wants you to take them long-term, discuss the downsides of these drugs, like the potentially increased risk of esophageal cancer. For more information on antacids and acid-suppressors, see Chapter 6.

- ▸ *Take medications with plenty of water,* and don't lie down after swallowing a pill. This helps it go down and stay down.

- ▸ *Consider an aspirin a day.* Early evidence suggests daily use of aspirin may dramatically cut the

For more information

International Foundation for Functional Gastrointestinal Disorders, Inc.
P.O. Box 170864
Milwaukee, WI 53217
888–964–2001 or
414–964–1799
www.iffgd.org

National Cancer Institute
National Institutes of Health
31 Center Drive
Building 31, Room 10A-19
Bethesda, MD 20892
800–4–CANCER or 800-422-6237
www.nci.nih.gov

risk of esophageal cancer. Discuss this treatment with your doctor before giving it a try.

Medical treatment options

Barrett's esophagus may or may not disappear with treatment. Some health experts recommend a follow-up Upper GI endoscopy every two to three years to make sure the condition has not become cancerous.

Doctors can also perform surgery and endoscopic procedures to help control GERD, but experts don't yet know whether surgery can slow the progression of Barrett's or prevent esophageal cancer. Lifestyle changes and medication are still the preferred treatments, but future therapies hold promise.

Experimental ablation therapies are being used to heal the esophagus by destroying or removing the abnormal Barrett's lining. There are three types of ablation therapy:

▸ *Photodynamic therapy,* which uses a modified laser.

▸ *Thermal ablation* burns off the Barrett's lining using heat.

▸ *Endoscopic mucosal resection* removes severely affected tissue and early cancer cells through an endoscope.

Hiatal hernia
Hidden cause of heartburn

You have a 60-percent chance of having a hiatal hernia if you're over age 60. The good news is, even if you have a hiatal hernia — no matter what your age — it's probably not a problem. You may not even know you have one.

That's because most hiatal hernias are small and don't cause any symptoms. When they do, it's usually only mild heartburn. Small hernias often go undetected until doctors find them while looking for something else. Large hiatal hernias, however, can become a problem.

What is a hiatal hernia?

It's a bulging of your stomach out of your abdominal cavity into your chest cavity. Your stomach normally stays beneath your diaphragm, a muscle that separates your chest cavity from your abdominal cavity. There's an opening, or hiatus, in the diaphragm where the esophagus comes through the abdominal wall and connects to your stomach. Where the stomach and esophagus connect, the lower esophageal sphincter (LES) muscle opens up to let food into your stomach, then closes to keep stomach contents from backing up into your esophagus.

When the opening gets weak or stretches, part of the stomach slips up through the diaphragm and bulges out. This bulge — a hiatal hernia — traps digestive materials and puts extra pressure on the

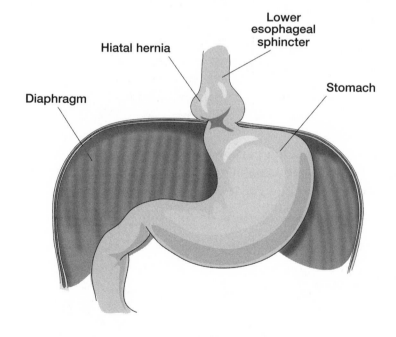

LES, which no longer has the diaphragm to help it stay shut. Chronic heartburn, or gastroesophageal reflux disease (GERD), may result as stomach acid creeps through the weakened LES and up into your esophagus.

Common symptoms and early warning signs

Doctors once thought hiatal hernias caused almost all reflux. They now think only large hiatal hernias may result in GERD and that many people with reflux problems don't actually have hiatal hernias.

Most hiatal hernias are sliding hernias, but occasionally part of the stomach forms a bulge alongside the esophagus known as a paraesophageal hernia. These can get twisted in a way that cuts off the blood supply and become dangerous. It's called strangulation and needs immediate medical attention.

Larger ones, however, can cause serious reflux and other major complications. When too much of the stomach pushes through, it puts pressure on the diaphragm, throat, and lungs. It can also create friction that causes lesions and bleeding.

Are you at risk?

Your risk of developing a hiatal hernia increases with age. Most occur in people over the age of 40, and women tend to get them more often than men.

Certain activities play a big part in causing hiatal hernias. Anything that puts too much pressure on your abdomen can contribute to hiatal hernia. For example:

▸ persistent or severe coughing or vomiting

▸ straining to go to the bathroom

▸ lifting heavy objects

▸ pregnancy or obesity

Medical procedures your doctor may order

Doctors usually find hiatal hernias by chance while looking for the cause of reflux, or chest or abdominal pain using one of these tests.

> **Barium swallow.** After you swallow barium, a liquid contrast dye, an X-ray machine may find the hernia sticking out near the bottom of the esophagus.

> **Upper GI endoscopy.** Thanks to throat anesthetic, your doctor can use a long, thin tube tipped with a tiny camera to see your esophagus — and any hernias — on a television monitor.

For more details about medical tests, see Chapter 7.

Nutritional defense against hiatal hernia

What and when you eat makes a difference in reflux symptoms caused by a hiatal hernia.

- ▸ **Citrus fruits and juices,** tomato products, and pepper can irritate a damaged esophageal lining.

- ▸ **Fatty foods, alcohol, chocolate,** and, especially, caffeine encourage reflux because they relax the LES muscle that keeps acid in your stomach.

- ▸ **Overeating makes your stomach overflow,** so several small meals are better than large ones.

- ▸ **Eating two or three hours before bedtime** gives food time to digest.

- ▸ **Sitting upright during and after meals** helps gravity move food quickly through your digestive system.

A roughage-rich diet may help you avoid developing a hiatal hernia. The straining that goes along with constipation is often blamed for causing this condition, and dietary fiber is a great help in staying regular. However, certain high-fiber foods, especially chunky, raw vegetables, may make your symptoms worse, so be careful what you eat.

Additional steps to take

The most likely trouble your hiatal hernia will cause is reflux and the heartburn that goes with it. This advice can help ease that discomfort.

▸ **Stop smoking.** Nicotine promotes reflux by relaxing the valve between your stomach and esophagus and, at the same time, stimulating the production of stomach acid.

▸ **Slim down to a healthy weight.** Being overweight puts extra pressure on your belly and squeezes stomach acid up into your esophagus.

▸ **Wear loose clothing.** Tight-fitting clothes and belts also put the squeeze on your stomach and force digestive juices into the esophagus.

▸ **Raise the head of your bed 6 to 9 inches.** Gravity helps keep stomach acid down where it belongs while you sleep.

▸ **Practice relaxation techniques,** such as deep breathing. Stress slows your digestion, which can make GERD worse.

▸ **Be careful about lifting,** straining, and other activities that put pressure on your diaphragm and abdominal cavity. They can cause or intensify a hiatal hernia, especially as you get older.

▸ **Stay alert for signs** that a hiatal hernia is getting bigger. If you know you have one and suffer severe chest pain, difficulty breathing, or trouble swallowing, get immediate medical attention.

Medical treatment options

No medicine will "cure" a hiatal hernia, but medication will help relieve the heartburn it can cause.

▸ **Antacids** neutralize stomach acid that gets into your esophagus.

▸ **H_2 blockers** reduce acid production by slowing down histamines. Stronger doses are available by prescription, but find out about side effects and interactions with other drugs.

▶ **_Proton pump inhibitors_** are the most effective drugs for GERD but also the most expensive. They work by directly blocking acid production.

Talk with your doctor before taking any drugs or discontinuing any medication.

Lifestyle adjustment and medicine to relieve the effects of GERD are the preferred treatments for hiatal hernia, but surgery may be appropriate in a few extreme cases, such as when:

▶ lifestyle adjustments and medication fail to control severe reflux.

▶ the hernia leads to chronic bleeding.

▶ the hernia blocks your esophagus.

Using either open or laparoscopic surgery, the surgeon will pull your stomach back into your abdomen and then fix the opening in your diaphragm. He may also do a fundoplication, where he wraps part of the stomach around the esophagus to support the LES muscle and prevent the stomach from slipping again.

GERD
Reverse reflux before it's too late

Stop popping antacids and get to your doctor if heartburn is a regular occurrence. You might have gastroesophageal reflux disease or GERD.

What is GERD?

When you eat, food travels down your esophagus into your stomach, which produces hydrochloric acid and other digestive juices. A valve at the top of your stomach, called the lower esophageal sphincter (LES), relaxes to let food in, then closes to seal out stomach acid.

The problem starts when the LES stops working properly, relaxing at the wrong time. Then, stomach acid washes up into your esophagus, an event called reflux.

A little reflux is normal. In fact, it can happen several times a day in healthy people without causing any symptoms or injury. But a growing number of people suffer from gastroesophageal reflux disease (GERD) — frequent reflux marked by severe symptoms, like heartburn, as well as damage to the esophagus, throat, or respiratory tract.

The stomach has a tough lining that protects it from its own digestive juices, but the esophagus doesn't. Frequent reflux can irritate, inflame, and damage the delicate lining of the esophagus.

Common symptoms and early warning signs

There's a good chance you have GERD if you experience heartburn more than twice a week. Along with more frequent heartburn, you may see symptoms like these.

- increased indigestion and regurgitation from your stomach
- difficulty swallowing or a feeling that food is trapped in your chest
- bleeding, including vomiting blood or having black or bloody bowel movements
- loss of appetite or unexplained weight loss

These warning signs are telling you to do something about your GERD before you suffer long-term damage. The more serious consequences are Barrett's esophagus and esophageal cancer.

You may also experience esophagitis, an inflammation of the esophagus, or esophageal stricture, a narrowing or blockage caused by inflammation and scar tissue. The stomach acid can also get into and damage organs connected to the esophagus, like the trachea (windpipe), larynx (voice box), and lungs.

Antacids and over-the-counter versions of prescription medicines may just cover up symptoms while GERD does more damage. If heartburn bothers you twice or more a week, see your doctor. He can find out if your esophagus is damaged and uncover the cause of your problems.

Are you at risk?

Several factors seem to raise your risk for GERD, although they don't necessarily cause it.

▶ *Obesity.* Being overweight can double your risk for GERD and related complications, including erosive esophagitis and esophageal cancer. The extra weight puts pressure on your stomach area, which can loosen the LES and force digestive juices into your esophagus.

▶ *Smoking.* Tobacco relaxes the LES, allowing stomach acid to creep up into your esophagus. Smoking also boosts acid production and decreases the saliva in your mouth, which might otherwise wash acid back out of your esophagus.

▶ *Alcohol.* Drinking alcoholic beverages also relaxes the LES, letting acid wash up into your esophagus.

▶ *Food.* What you eat can have a huge impact on heartburn symptoms. Coffee, chocolate, fatty foods, peppermint, sodas, and acidic foods, such as oranges and tomatoes, can aggravate GERD. Different foods may bother different people.

▶ *Slow digestion.* Some people experience "delayed gastric emptying," which means food stays in their stomach longer than normal. Slow digestion can cause heartburn.

GERD may contribute to conditions outside the esophagus including:

▶ hoarse voice

▶ chronic cough

▶ erosion of tooth enamel

▶ lung disease

▶ breathing difficulty in people who have asthma

▸ *Hiatal hernia.* In some people, part of the stomach bulges through the opening in the diaphragm, crowding the esophagus. This kind of hernia can lead to GERD, though not all people with hiatal hernias have GERD.

▸ *Family history.* Your risk for GERD is higher if one of your parents suffered with it.

Medical procedures your doctor may order

Your symptoms will probably tell your doctor you have GERD, but he may confirm or expand his diagnosis with one or more of these tests.

▸ *Upper GI endoscopy.* Thanks to a throat anesthetic, your doctor can scrutinize your esophagus for inflammation and erosion with a long, thin tube tipped with a tiny camera. If she finds trouble, she can snip a tiny amount of tissue and have it analyzed, called a biopsy, to find out whether GERD is the culprit.

▸ *Barium swallow.* After you swallow barium, a liquid contrast dye, a special X-ray machine makes moving X-rays to show whether the barium backs up into your esophagus after entering your stomach.

▸ *Esophageal manometry.* A long, thin tube with a pressure sensor can measure the pressure of your lower esophageal sphincter (LES.) Although this valve should keep stomach acid from escaping into your esophagus, the LES pressure might be too low to prevent it.

▸ *Esophageal pH test.* A data recorder and a pH probe — a thin tube with a tiny pH meter at the end — monitor the acidity in your esophagus for 24-hours. If your symptoms match up to episodes of high acidity, you probably have GERD.

For more details about medical tests, see Chapter 7.

Nutritional defense against GERD

Take a close look at what you're eating. With GERD, you'll probably get better results cutting out foods and drinks that trigger the condition than to try and find foods to make it better.

Most importantly, start cutting fatty foods out of your diet. They cause the stomach to empty slower, so food and acid stick around longer. They also trigger a chemical change that relaxes the LES, letting acid wash up into your esophagus.

Other prime candidates for elimination include:

▸ chocolate, garlic, onions, and greasy or spicy foods.

▸ highly acidic foods, such as citrus fruit and juices and tomato products.

▸ alcohol, caffeine, or carbonated beverages.

▸ pepper, spearmint, peppermint, mustard, and vinegar.

The same things don't bother everyone. If you suspect a certain food or beverage is contributing to your problem, stay away from it for several days and see if you feel better. Then notice what happens when you start eating or drinking it again.

Try following these general rules to put a cap on GERD.

▸ *Eat more low-acid fruits and vegetables* and less high-fat meat and fried food. You can also eat more whole-grain foods to absorb extra stomach acid.

▸ *Avoid overeating.* Large meals increase acid production, and a full stomach is more likely to overflow into the esophagus.

▸ *Skip processed meats.* They contain nitrates, chemicals that may increase the risk of esophageal cancer in people with GERD and those taking acid-suppressing medications.

▸ *Drink water throughout the day in small amounts.* Drinking too much at one time could distend your stomach and increase your heartburn. Six to eight 8-ounce glasses should help your digestion. Water washes acid out of your esophagus and dilutes the acid in your stomach. But don't drink liquids with meals since you need stomach acid to digest your food. An hour before or after is best.

Additional steps to take

Your best defense against GERD is to practice healthy habits that relieve heartburn.

▸ **Quit smoking and avoid alcohol.** Both loosen the LES and tend to cause reflux.

▸ **Slim down to a healthy weight.** Being overweight puts the squeeze on your stomach and abdomen and may cause the LES to relax.

▸ **Stay away from foods that stimulate reflux,** such as chocolate, spicy food, tomato sauce, orange juice, peppermint, onions, and soft drinks.

▸ **Control nighttime eating.** Don't lie down for at least two hours after eating, and don't eat again for at least two hours before bedtime. This gives stomach acid a chance to decrease before you lie down.

▸ **Wear clothes and belts** that fit comfortably around your stomach. Don't wear anything tight.

▸ **Sit up straight when you eat.** Never stand, lie down, or bend over after eating. This forces food and stomach acid back up into your esophagus.

▸ **Raise the head of your bed** about 6 inches by placing blocks under your bedposts, or slide a sleeping wedge under your mattress. This lets gravity keep the contents of your stomach out of your esophagus while you sleep.

▸ **Avoid heavy lifting and straining.** This causes your abdominal muscles to contract and squeeze stomach acid into your esophagus.

Medical treatment options

Your first line of defense against GERD is cheap, nonprescription liquids or tablets that stop your stomach from making acid. These include H$_2$ blockers, like Tagamet, Pepcid, and Zantac.

If you need something stronger, your doctor may prescribe drugs called proton-pump inhibitors (PPIs). The PPI Prevacid is also available in an inexpensive, over-the-counter, nonprescription strength.

Promotility agents, like Reglan, may be prescribed along with acid-reducing medications. They work by strengthening your LES and encouraging your stomach to empty faster. For more information, please see *Antacids* in Chapter 6.

Lifestyle changes and medication are the more preferred and proven treatments for GERD. Surgery and endoscopic procedures are newer alternatives, but their long-term effectiveness is still being determined.

▸ Fundoplication is the most common surgery for GERD. A surgeon lifts up part of the stomach, wraps it around the lower esophagus, and sews it into place so it adds strength to the lower esophageal sphincter (LES) muscle. This surgery can be done using a laparoscope, allowing for small incisions and less time in the hospital.

▸ You can also undergo a newer procedure called endoscopic gastroplication, where the surgeon stitches a "pleat" that narrows the opening between your stomach and esophagus. This procedure requires no

For a good night's rest, sleep on your left side to reduce acid reflux. That's because your esophagus angles a bit to the left where it connects to your stomach. Lying on your right side increases the tilt and acid can drip out of your stomach. But if you lie on your left side, the acid has an uphill climb. Try a sleeping wedge behind your back to keep you facing left so you can sleep in peace.

incisions, general anesthesia, or hospital stays. It also costs less than fundoplication.

▸ Other endoscopic procedures involve injections or the creation of scar tissue to strengthen the LES. These methods can have serious side effects and are still being studied.

For more information

National Heartburn Alliance
877-471-2081
www.heartburnalliance.org

An operation may not be the best answer to your GERD problems. Surgery can cause unpleasant symptoms, like bloating, diarrhea, excessive gas, and difficulty swallowing. With any surgery, there is always the risk of serious, even fatal, complications. What's more, about a third of the people who have laparoscopic fundoplication still have to take medicine.

Talk with your doctor before taking any drugs or discontinuing any medication.

Gastritis
Uncover causes of stomach pain

Ouch! That pain in your stomach could be more than just a tummy ache. You could have gastritis, a catchall term for several conditions involving inflammation of your stomach lining. It also has several possible causes.

What causes gastritis?

The most common cause worldwide is infection by *Helicobacter pylori*, or *H. pylori*, the same bacteria responsible for most ulcers and most cases of stomach cancer. In fact, gastritis can lead to ulcers and more serious symptoms.

Frequent use of nonsteroidal anti-inflammatory drugs (NSAIDs), such as aspirin and ibuprofen, can also spark gastritis. Certain diseases, like pernicious anemia and autoimmune disorders, can also cause it. Smoking or drinking too much alcohol can trigger gastritis. It can also develop after major surgery, serious injury, burns, or severe infections.

H. pylori infections, the most common cause of gastritis, afflict approximately two-thirds of the world's population at one time or another. If left untreated, these infections can lead to ulcers, as well as stomach cancer.

Common symptoms and early warning signs

If you have abdominal pain, upset stomach, and indigestion, you may have gastritis. You could also experience belching, bloating, nausea, vomiting, and a feeling of fullness or burning in your upper abdomen. On the other hand, you may not have any symptoms, just an inflamed stomach lining, that could lead to future problems.

Blood in your vomit or black stools could signal stomach bleeding, a very serious consequence of gastritis and associated ulcers that may be free of other symptoms. See your doctor right away.

Are you at risk?

Your odds of getting gastritis may go up if any of these apply to you.

- ▶ You often drink alcohol or caffeine-rich beverages or eat irritating foods, like hot peppers and other spicy foods.
- ▶ You've used nonsteroidal anti-inflammatory drugs (NSAIDs), such as aspirin or ibuprofen, for a long time.
- ▶ You're infected with *H. pylori* bacteria.
- ▶ You have food or drink allergies.
- ▶ You have pernicious anemia, kidney disease, diabetes, or an autoimmune problem.

> ▸ You have a chronic reflux of bile, bile acids, or pancreatic juices from the uppermost part of your small intestine back into your stomach.

Medical procedures your doctor may order

These tests may help uncover the source of your gastritis.

Upper gastrointestinal endoscopy. Your doctor can see the inflammation of gastritis in your stomach using a camera-tipped tube. She may also remove a tiny tissue sample from your stomach lining so it can be analyzed to find the cause of your gastritis.

Blood test. A simple blood test can check for anemia, or low red blood cell count. Bleeding from the stomach can cause anemia.

Stool test. A fecal occult blood test (FOBT) checks for blood in your stool. This may be a symptom of bleeding in your digestive tract, possibly in your stomach. Another stool test — the *H. pylori* stool antigen test — checks for traces of a substance that appears when ulcer-causing *H. pylori* bacteria have infected your digestive tract.

Breath test. If drinking a special mixture adds more carbon to your breath, you probably have infection by *H. pylori*.

For more details about medical tests, see Chapter 7.

A new pilot study suggests that *H. pylori* may be more common in people who have atrial fibrillation, a heart rhythm disturbance, than in people who don't have it. Taking antibiotics to get rid of *H. pylori* may help reduce atrial fibrillation, but more research is needed to confirm the link.

Nutritional defense against gastritis

Eating certain foods and avoiding others is a big part of managing gastritis.

- ▸ **Learn to love these four foods**, green tea, plantains, yogurt, and unprocessed honey, to ease inflammation and prevent flare-ups.

- ▸ **Stay away from foods that may irritate your stomach.** Citrus fruits, tomatoes, soda, orange juice, caffeine, alcohol, spicy foods, fried or fatty foods, and milk often spell trouble.

Additional steps to take

When it comes to gastritis, how and when you eat can be just as important as what you eat. Besides avoiding irritating, high-acid foods, take the following steps to foil gastritis.

- ▸ **Eat several small meals** throughout the day. This is gentler on your digestive system than three large meals.

- ▸ **Drink plenty of water.** It's better to drink liquids between meals rather than with meals.

- ▸ **Don't eat less than four hours** before bedtime.

A new study suggests that sulforaphane — a powerful compound in broccoli sprouts — might help ease gastritis. In the study, 40 people ate around 3 1/2 ounces of either broccoli sprouts or alfalfa sprouts every day for two months. Alfalfa sprouts have almost no sulforaphane but are very similar to broccoli sprouts. The broccoli sprouts stopped H. pylori from setting up colonies and reduced the symptoms of gastritis, while the alfalfa sprouts did not. You can buy BroccoSprouts, a product developed by Johns Hopkins University researchers, at many food stores. For more information about their products, including Brassica tea, call toll-free 877-747-1277 or visit www.brassica.com.

- ▸ **Engage in regular physical activity,** like walking or swimming.

- ▸ **Eat fiber-rich foods,** like fruits, veggies, and oat bran. A fiber supplement, like Metamucil, might help, too.

For years, many doctors said they were crazy, but the scientists who discovered the link between stomach ulcers, gastritis, stomach cancer, and *H. pylori* bacteria proved them wrong when they won the 2005 Nobel Prize for Medicine. Since Australians Barry Marshall and Robin Warren made their discovery, the FDA has approved eight variations of their antibiotic-based treatment for ulcers.

▸ *Load up on vitamin C-rich fruits and veggies,* like strawberries, broccoli, cantaloupe, Brussels sprouts, and sweet peppers.

Medical treatment options

Your doctor may prescribe or suggest medicines like these to help you.

▸ Some doctors may treat minor gastritis with acid reducers, but two weeks of a two-antibiotic combo may be necessary to get rid of infections with *H. pylori,* the culprit behind most cases of gastritis, as well as ulcers and stomach cancer. Dr. Marshall, the Nobel prize winner, recommends amoxicillin and clarithromycin (Biaxin). Other effective combos include metronidazole (Flagyl) and clarithromycin, as well as metronidazole and tetracycline. The antibiotics may be combined with other drugs, like bismuth and acid reducers.

▸ Bismuth subsalicylate, the active ingredient in Pepto-Bismol and Bismatrol, protects your stomach lining and helps kill *H. pylori.* It's a good alternative if your doctor is ignorant about the link between gastritis, ulcers, stomach cancer, and *H. pylori* infection, but you may need to take it for a longer period than prescription antibiotics. Just remember that bismuth-based products contain around 1 gram of salicylates for every four tablets so be sure to cut back on other salicylate-containing medication, including aspirin, while taking bismuth.

▸ To promote healing and ease your discomfort, you may take drugs that inhibit acid production — histamine-2 (H_2) blockers, such as cimetidine (Tagamet), famotidine (Pepcid), ranitidine

(Zantac) or proton pump inhibitors, such as esomeprazole (Nexium), lansoprazole (Prevacid), and omeprazole (Prilosec).

▸ Taking antacids can also relieve your symptoms and help promote healing.

▸ Sucralfate helps prevent irritation and promote healing, but it doesn't have any effect on acid production.

Stay away from aspirin and other nonsteroidal anti-inflammatory drugs, like ibuprofen, that might irritate your stomach lining. Arthritis formulas can be especially hard on your stomach. If you need a pain reliever, acetaminophen may be your best bet.

Talk with your doctor before taking any drugs or discontinuing any medication.

Peptic ulcers
Find out what's eating you

You may think only people who have high-stress lifestyles get peptic ulcers, but that's not the case. Anybody can get one.

What is a peptic ulcer?

A peptic ulcer is a sore on the lining of your stomach or duodenum, the first part of the small intestine. Stomach ulcers are also called gastric ulcers, while intestinal ulcers are called duodenal ulcers. Ulcers usually are the size of a pencil eraser or smaller, but their symptoms can make you miserable.

Most people once thought peptic ulcers were caused by stress or spicy foods. But in the 1980s, Australians Barry Marshall and Robin Warren made an amazing discovery — one that later won them the 2005 Nobel Prize. They uncovered the most treatable cause of ulcers, *Helicobacter pylori* (*H. pylori*), a corkscrew-shaped bacterium and the

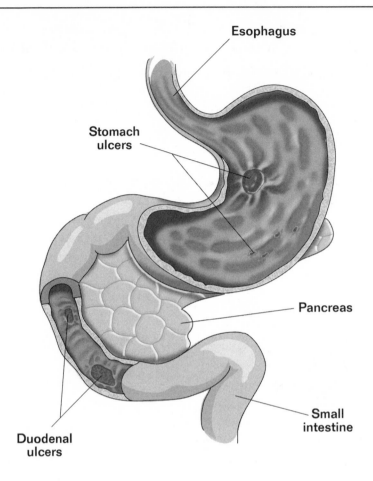

Esophagus

Stomach
ulcers

Pancreas

Small
intestine

Duodenal
ulcers

only known bacterium that can live in the lining of the stomach and set up colonies.

Your stomach and small intestine are protected from acidic gastric juice by a special lining, which produces mucus that protects your stomach. Infection by *H. pylori* weakens this protective lining and allows gastric juice to eat into your stomach or small intestine, creating a painful ulcer. The good news is these ulcers can be treated with antibiotics and, in most cases, cured.

Then again, most, but not all, peptic ulcers are caused by bacteria. They can also result from the regular use of nonsteroidal anti-inflammatory drugs (NSAIDs), like aspirin and ibuprofen. Because they block enzymes that help protect the lining of your gut, NSAIDs quadruple your risk of getting an ulcer, especially a stomach ulcer.

Common symptoms and early warning signs

Heartburn and abdominal discomfort are key symptoms of both stomach and duodenal ulcers. But a tomach ulcer is more likely to cause weight loss, particularly if eating triggers pain or makes it worse.

The pain from duodenal ulcers usually occurs between meals and in the middle of the night. Eating may ease the pain so you're more likely to gain weight. Nausea, vomiting, and loss of appetite are also ulcer symptoms, but they're less common.

Are you at risk?

Small intestine or duodenal ulcers are more common than gastric, or stomach, ulcers. Men are more likely to get duodenal ulcers, while women are more prone to gastric ulcers. In fact, duodenal ulcers are twice as common in men and occur more frequently in people ages 30 to 50. Gastric ulcers are more common in people over age 60.

Medical procedures your doctor may order

Symptoms of gastritis or ulcers can be treated by a simple, two-week regimen of antibiotics without testing for *H. pylori*. However, your doctor might use these tests to help him make a diagnosis:

Blood test to detect H. pylori. A laboratory can check a sample of your blood for antibodies to *H. pylori* bacteria. That's a sure sign of the bacteria, and you'll keep producing those antibodies years after your *H. pylori* has been wiped out.

Breath test to detect H. pylori. At your doctor's office, you'll drink a urea liquid containing special carbon atoms. *H. pylori* break down the liquid, which releases the carbon. If the breath analyzer finds higher-than-normal carbon amounts in your breath, you are infected with *H. pylori*.

Stool test. You provide a stool sample, and the lab checks it for antigens produced in response to *H. pylori*.

Without treatment, peptic ulcers can lead to complications, like bleeding or holes, in your stomach or small intestine. If scarring occurs, it could even close up the opening to your stomach, leaving surgery as your only choice.

Barium swallow. After drinking barium, a liquid contrast dye, you have X-rays of your stomach and small intestine taken. If you have an ulcer, the X-rays may show your doctor where it's lurking.

Upper GI endoscopy. Your doctor uses a long, thin tube with a tiny camera attached to check your stomach and duodenum for ulcers. You'll be given throat anesthetic, a sedative, or painkillers before the tube is inserted. Instruments inserted through the tube can take a tiny pinch of tissue, called a biopsy, so a lab can check it for *H. pylori*. This is the test of choice for stomach ulcers because they should always be biopsied for cancer.

For more details about medical tests, see Chapter 7.

Nutritional defense against peptic ulcers

Some foods help protect you from peptic ulcers. Try these healthy suggestions. Your stomach will thank you.

- ▶ *Discover the power of broccoli.* Eating broccoli products, like broccoli sprouts, helps clear up infectious gastritis caused by *H. pylori* infection. Future studies may also show a benefit in helping ulcers heal, but this is yet to be proven.

- ▶ *Enjoy a spoonful of honey* to get sweet relief from ulcer pain. Honey acts as an antibacterial, and research shows it zooms in on *H. pylori.* To help soothe your discomfort, eat a tablespoon of honey an hour before meals and at bedtime.

▸ ***Add pizzazz with garlic.*** This fragrant bulb also acts as an anti-bacterial. A Dutch study found that garlic slowed the growth of four different strains of *H. pylori* in the lab.

▸ ***Use olive oil instead of butter,*** and you might give your stomach an added boost of protection. Polyunsaturated fats, like olive oil, fish oil, and sunflower oil, prevented the growth of *H. pylori* in laboratory tests.

▸ ***Eat more cranberries.*** Just as they protect your urinary tract from bacterial infections, cranberries could also protect your stomach lining from *H. pylori* and prevent an ulcer from forming.

▸ ***Snack on yogurt.*** *Lactobacillus casei*, a "friendly" bacteria found in some yogurt products, such as DanActive, destroyed *H. pylori* in test tube studies.

▸ ***Visit the produce aisle.*** Researchers recently discovered that fiber from fruits and vegetables could reduce your risk of ulcers. Fiber seems to encourage the growth of the protective mucous lining.

Additional steps to take

You can protect yourself from peptic ulcers by picking up some good habits and breaking some bad ones.

Researchers at Johns Hopkins School of Medicine discovered that broccoli contains disease-fighting phytochemicals. The most powerful of these phytochemicals is sulforaphane, which stimulates protective enzymes that help protect you from cancer. Sulforaphane also has antibiotic powers that kill some bacteria, like *H. pylori*. Broccoli products, including BroccoSprouts and Brassica tea, are proven to have the most powerful antibiotic effect compared to other nutritional products. For more information, call toll-free 877-747-1277 or visit www.brassica.com. Also, see *Broccoli sprouts* in Chapter 5.

▶ **Wash your hands before meals** and after using the restroom. This will help prevent the spread of *H. pylori*. And don't kiss anyone on the mouth who may have infectious gastritis or ulcers caused by *H. pylori*.

▶ **Avoid NSAIDs.** If you take nonsteroidal anti-inflammatory drugs (NSAIDs), like aspirin and ibuprofen, on a regular basis, discuss alternative medications with your doctor. Some health experts say 4 grams of acetaminophen a day can give the same pain relief for osteoarthritis as ibuprofen, without the risk of ulcers. If your doctor advises taking aspirin to help prevent a heart attack, taking one or two low-dose, 81 mg enteric-coated aspirin a day has less risk of causing ulcers than taking other forms. Also, tell your doctor if you have an ulcer, history of ulcers, or concerns about developing an ulcer.

▶ **Reach for an antacid.** Over-the-counter antacids help ease stomach pain if you already have an ulcer. Bismuth subsalicylate also helps. It's an ingredient in Pepto-Bismol that protects your stomach lining and helps heal your ulcer by killing *H. pylori* bacteria along with prescription antibiotics.

▶ **Learn ways to manage stress.** Give your ulcer the chance to heal by learning to deal with stress. This keeps your stomach from making too much stomach acid.

▶ **Avoid drinking alcohol.** Alcoholic beverages can irritate your stomach.

▶ **Stop smoking.** Smoking keeps ulcers from healing and may cause them to come back again after they heal.

Medical treatment options

Your doctor could prescribe a combination of drugs to treat your ulcer.

▶ For ulcers caused by bacteria, antibiotics are the most effective treatment. They can cure 80 to 90 percent of peptic ulcers. Taking a combination of prescription antibiotics, like amoxicillin and clarithromycin (Biaxin) or tetracycline and metronidazole, which are also very effective although metronidazole may have potentially greater side effects, and nonprescription bismuth subsalicylate (Pepto-Bismol) for up to four weeks seems to work best.

▸ H$_2$ blockers, like cimetidine (Tagamet), famotidine (Pepcid), and ranitidine (Zantac), and proton pump inhibitors, such as esomeprazole (Nexium), lansoprazole (Prevacid), and omeprazole (Prilosec), reduce stomach acid and help your ulcer to heal. This treatment should be the first choice for noninfectious ulcers caused by taking aspirin or other NSAID regularly. Yet, keep in mind that some health experts are concerned that the long-term use of these medications might raise your risk of esophageal cancer. See your doctor regularly and talk with him about this concern.

Talk with your doctor before taking any drugs or discontinuing any medication.

Researchers in Poland say grapefruit extract can help heal peptic ulcers. The extract, taken from the fruit's seeds, is an antibacterial and an antioxidant, which calms the digestive tract and helps the healing process.

Crohn's disease
Protect your immune system from attack

President Dwight D. Eisenhower was diagnosed with Crohn's disease during his first term in office. But that didn't stop him from winning re-election and running the country for another four years. Crohn's doesn't have to stop you either. Build up your knowledge of this condition so you can find ways to help yourself and manage your symptoms.

What is Crohn's disease?

Crohn's disease (CD) is a chronic condition that can affect your entire digestive system, but it usually targets the intestines. Somehow, Crohn's disease is a consequence of an immune system gone haywire.

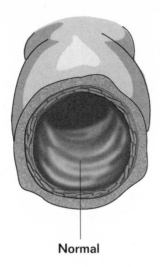 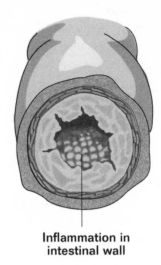

Normal

Inflammation in
intestinal wall

Something triggers inflammation in the walls of your small intestine, your large intestine, or both. And the next thing you know, you've got crampy abdominal pain and frequent diarrhea.

Like a forest fire, Crohn's may sear some parts of your intestines while leaving others untouched. What's more, it may alternate between flare-ups with raging symptoms and calm periods when symptoms die down. CD isn't contagious, and it is treatable. Unfortunately, it doesn't have a cure — at least not yet, but there are interesting dietary approaches that may help keep it in check and prevent flare-ups.

Crohn's is considered an IBD or inflammatory bowel disease. CD and its evil twin, ulcerative colitis, are considered IBDs because both may cause inflammation in your colon.

Your doctor may also refer to CD as ileitis, colitis, ileocolitis, or jejunoileitis. These terms tell which parts of your intestines are inflamed, and that may determine the symptoms and complications you're most likely to experience.

About 20 percent of the people with CD have colitis, meaning only the large intestine is affected. Between 30 and 40 percent have either ileitis or jejunoileitis, where the small intestine is inflamed, but not the colon. Another 30 to 40 percent have ileocolitis, or CD affecting both the small and large intestines. CD may sometimes affect other areas of the digestive tract, even the esophagus.

Common symptoms and early warning signs

Reaching a Crohn's diagnosis can take years of testing because Crohn's symptoms resemble those of other diseases, like ileal tuberculosis, ulcerative colitis, and lymphoma. What's more, the early symptoms of Crohn's may also be diagnosed as appendicitis, especially if there's lower-right abdominal pain. That's why knowing Crohn's other characteristics, including the ones that have no obvious link to the digestive system, is important.

The most common early symptoms are abdominal cramps, chronic diarrhea — sometimes bloody, and weight loss. Other symptoms include nausea, loss of appetite, fever, and bleeding from the rectum. The following complications and symptoms may also develop.

▶ arthritis

▶ fatigue

▶ unusual skin problems

▶ inflammation in the eyes or mouth

▶ dehydration

▶ kidney stones

▶ gallstones

▶ inflammation of the spine or pelvic joints

Doctors may soon have new ways to treat CD, thanks to the latest research. Scientists say your small intestine casts off old cells from its walls, but quickly repairs the area where the cells were. Now, new animal research suggests that this automatic repair may not happen in people with Crohn's — leaving gaps where bacteria can sneak in and start trouble. More research is coming soon, so stay tuned.

▸ blockage or narrowing in the intestine

▸ vitamin and mineral deficiencies

▸ malnutrition caused by problems absorbing fats, protein, and carbohydrates

▸ abscesses or pockets of infection filled with pus

▸ tunnels, called fistulas, that develop between the intestine and other organs or between the intestine and the skin

Are you at risk?

Also, remember that you're more likely to have Crohn's if you have other risk factors for the disease, so be sure to mention these characteristics to your doctor.

▸ **Family history.** Someone else in your family has some form of Crohn's disease or another IBD.

▸ **Age.** You're under the age of 35 or between the ages of 50 and 70.

Scientists still aren't sure what causes Crohn's. Research suggests that genetics may contribute to some cases. Scientists also suspect that a virus or bacterium may play a role, too. Researchers are constantly hunting for both the causes and a cure.

Medical procedures your doctor may order

Crohn's disease often resembles several other conditions. After a comprehensive physical exam, these tests can help your doctor make a correct diagnosis.

Stool sample. A laboratory checks the stool sample you provide for hidden blood. Intestinal bleeding from CD is one possible source of blood.

Blood tests. Blood tests show signs of inflammation, like increased white blood cell count, high C-reactive protein, or something called an elevated erythrocyte sedimentation rate (ESR). A low red blood cell count (anemia) might mean bleeding in your colon.

Barium swallow. You're given a barium drink to help X-rays reveal inflammation or other signs of CD in the small intestine. The small bowel series is part of the barium swallow in which barium coats the small intestine. Enteroclysis, a variation on the small bowel series, has a greater risk of side effects but may uncover small areas of possible cancer. The doctor gives you a mild anesthetic and inserts a tube through your mouth down into your intestine. Barium pumped through the tube helps the small intestine show up more clearly on X-rays.

Double-contrast barium enema. For extra detail on X-rays, air is put into your colon, and you're given an enema with barium. This may reveal a thickened colon wall, nodules, or other signs of Crohn's.

Colonoscopy. With help from anesthesia and painkillers, your doctor can use a long tube tipped with a camera to look inside your colon for inflammation or bleeding from CD.

Biopsy. Instruments passed through the colonoscopy tube can take a tiny tissue sample from inside the colon. Analysis of the sample may help diagnose or rule out Crohn's.

Ultrasound. As a handheld ultrasound "scanner" is drawn over your abdominal area, a sonar-like device creates images with sound waves. This scan can find fistulas or abscesses.

Computed tomography (CT) scan. This scan may show signs of Crohn's, like fistulas, outside the colon and small intestine. It may also be used to tell which inflammatory bowel disease you may have — CD or ulcerative colitis.

New research suggests you may also have a higher risk of asthma, bronchitis, arthritis, psoriasis, and multiple sclerosis if you have inflammatory bowel disease.

If you have inflammatory bowel disease, your symptoms and the condition of your intestines may prevent you from taking some of these tests.

For more details about medical tests, see Chapter 7.

Experimental treatment promising

A bold, experimental treatment helped some Crohn's sufferers shed their symptoms, using medicines already approved by the Food and Drug Administration (FDA). What's more, this new treatment may hint at why some people develop Crohn's in the first place.

A few researchers suggest that Crohn's may come from the same microbe as Johne's disease, a cattle disease with similar symptoms. Bacteria called *mycobacterium avium paratuberculosis* (MAP), which cows may pass along in their milk, cause Johne's disease. MAP might also be able to sneak into lakes and streams near herds, a possible express route into local water supplies.

Although this theory isn't proven, it could open up new options for anyone who has Crohn's or is concerned about getting it. At least one researcher suggests that milk should be ultra-pasteurized before you

Inflammatory bowel disease at a glance	
Crohn's disease	**Ulcerative colitis**
usually affects the small intestine but entire digestive tract can be involved	affects the colon, rectum, and, in rare cases, the small intestine
inflames all the layers of the intestinal wall	only inflames the top layer of the colon's lining
rectal bleeding or blood in the stool may occur	bleeding or blood in the stool occurs often

drink it. That means the milk must be heated to 280 degrees Fahrenheit or higher for at least two seconds to destroy all disease-producing bacteria and viruses, including MAP, which is incompletely killed by ordinary low-temperature pasteurization. If you want to try ultra-pasteurized milk, look for containers with "ultra-pasteurized" on the label.

But that's not the only new possibility. Some scientists have asked this question — if MAP causes some, or perhaps most, cases of CD, as some researchers think, could MAP-fighting antibiotics stop Crohn's symptoms? Small studies suggest they might. Combining rifabutin with antibiotics like clarithromycin or clofazimine appears to wipe out Crohn's symptoms for some and brings significant relief to others. In fact, some people in the studies were able to cut back on their CD medicines — or even stop taking them.

But don't forget these studies are preliminary, and this therapy won't be right for everyone. Some study participants couldn't tolerate the medicines and others saw no improvement. Even those whose Crohn's symptoms got better struggled with drug side effects, like fatigue, joint pain, yellowing or reddening of the skin, lower white blood cell count, and increased liver enzymes.

A new study suggests that a cancer drug called sargramostim — trade name Leukine — could help some Crohn's sufferers ease their symptoms, or even get rid of them. In a small, six-week study, 48 percent of those taking the drug saw improvement in their symptoms, while only 26 percent of those taking a placebo saw an improvement. Past research has suggested CD is the result of an immune system in overdrive, so doctors have prescribed immune-suppressing drugs. But this medicine revs up the immune system, making some scientists wonder if Crohn's might be caused by aspects of the immune system that don't reach full power.

Yet, if this antibiotic therapy can be proven safe and effective for most people, it might offer months of relief to many Crohn's sufferers. Stay tuned to see what the clinical trials and research reveal.

Try something different. Bismuth subsalicylate (Pepto-Bismol) may also be helpful in treating Crohn's. Some victims of the disease, like Peggy Fleming, the ice skating champion, declare that taking it regularly keeps them free of symptoms. There is a rationale for how it might work. Bismuth subsalicylate kills the *H. pylori* bacteria that drill into the lining of the stomach and cause gastritis and ulcers. It seems plausible that it might also help kill MAP bacteria that are thought to hide in the intestinal wall and trigger Crohn's disease. This theory may also apply to sulforaphane in broccoli products. For more information about BroccoSprouts and Brassica teas, call toll-free 877-747-1277 or visit *www.brassica.com*. However, there are no scientific studies yet that have investigated this hypothesis.

Up to 40 percent of people with Crohn's can't properly absorb carbohydrates. So foods like bread and potatoes lead to gas, bloating, diarrhea, and lost nutrients. If carbohydrates trouble you, ask your doctor what to do.

Nutritional defense against Crohn's disease

What you eat won't cause Crohn's, but wise choices can help soothe your symptoms.

▶ *Eat smaller meals* more frequently.

▶ **Avoid foods** that aggravate your symptoms. Milk, alcohol, and hot spices are common culprits. Keep a food diary to spot foods that give you trouble.

▶ *Cut back on greasy foods,* fried foods, and caffeine to help prevent diarrhea, cramping, and gas.

▶ *Eliminate milk and milk products* if you're lactose-intolerant, or think you might be, especially since recent research implicates a bacterium often found in milk as a suspected trigger of many cases of Crohn's.

▶ **Ask your doctor** about temporarily switching to a low-fiber, low-residue diet if you have narrowing of the intestine. Avoid intestine-rattling foods, like raw fruits, raw vegetables, nuts, and seeds. However, soluble fiber, like pectin, may slow the passage of food through the intestines and help relieve some symptoms of Crohn's.

▶ **Try lactobacillus supplements** or live culture yogurt. The new DanActive cultured dairy drink from Dannon may be especially helpful in many digestive conditions.

▶ **Talk with your doctor about folic acid** supplements if he has prescribed methotrexate, a powerful immune system suppressor that blocks the action of folic acid. According to the American College of Gastroenterology, folic acid should be taken with methotrexate to decrease some side effects. Potential side effects and risks include nausea, vomiting, infections, suppressed bone marrow, and liver inflammation.

▶ **Consider supplements.** Ask a doctor who specializes in the treatment of Crohn's disease which vitamin and mineral deficiencies are possible and whether you should take nutritional supplements. But watch out for vitamin D side effects, especially if you're over 55. Vitamin D deficiency is one of

Bacteria aren't always bad. In fact, some can be quite good — like *E. coli*. Usually, you want to avoid *E. coli*, a bacterium that can cause serious infection. But one particular strain, *Escherichia coli* (*E. coli*) Nissle 1917, sold under the brand name Mutaflor, helps maintain remission in inflammatory bowel diseases, like Crohn's disease and ulcerative colitis. It has worked as safely and effectively as the anti-inflammatory drug mesalamine for ulcerative colitis and better than placebo in Crohn's. In fact, only one-third of the people on Mutaflor in a recent study had a relapse of Crohn's disease, compared to two-thirds on placebo. For more information, see *Ulcerative colitis* in this chapter and *Probiotics* in Chapter 4.

the most common nutritional deficiencies in people with CD, but talk with your doctor before taking supplements. People 55 or older are more likely to experience bad reactions or side effects. Symptoms from vitamin D supplements may include nausea, vomiting, abnormal thirst, increased urination, headache, irritability, weakness, and depression. Ask your doctor what to do if these symptoms occur.

▶ *Reduce inflammation.* Check with your doctor about taking fish oil supplements and probiotic supplements. Fish oil has anti-inflammatory properties that might help people with CD, without the long-term side effects of the prescription anti-inflammatory drugs called corticosteroids. A study of people with Crohn's disease showed that those who took low-dose fish-oil capsules for a year had fewer relapses than those who didn't. Fish oil seemed to have this effect because it kept inflammation from flaring up. Zinc supplements or flaxseed oil in food or supplements also may help reduce inflammation. Some experts even think people with CD could benefit from increasing their intake of antioxidant vitamins, such as vitamins E and C.

For more information

Two heads may be better than one when it comes to managing Crohn's. Take advantage of a support group to help you cope with this challenging disease.

Crohn's & Colitis Foundation of America, Inc.
386 Park Avenue South,
17th Floor
New York, NY 10016-8804
800-932-2423
www.ccfa.org

Additional steps to take

Until a cure is found for Crohn's, your best bet is to prevent inflammation and control your symptoms. Start with these tips.

▶ *Learn how to care for yourself* and how to manage any controllable aspects of Crohn's. The American Gastroenterological Association suggests getting familiar with how Crohn's affects you.

▶ *Ask your doctor about medications,* like antidiarrheals, to help soothe your symptoms.

▶ *Stop* smoking.

▶ *Consider screenings.* Ask your doctor whether you need screenings for osteoporosis, anemia, colon cancer, or other conditions linked with Crohn's.

▶ *Learn ways* to manage stress.

▶ *Avoid NSAIDS,* like ibuprofen and aspirin, unless you take them to prevent serious conditions, like heart attack or stroke. Ask your doctor which painkillers are safe for you.

Medical treatment options

Always keep learning about your treatment options so you'll make sound decisions. Here are two hot new options, as well as an old standby some people may eventually need to consider.

▶ *Anti-interleukin-12* injections help prevent an immune system reaction that leads to inflammation.

▶ *Trichuris suis* is an experimental treatment using a type of harmless-to-humans pig whipworm egg supplement that has been shown to put a damper on the immune reactions that ignite CD symptoms. This pig whipworm egg therapy was pioneered by University of Iowa gastroenterologist Joel Weinstock and his colleagues. For more information, see *Pig whipworm egg therapy* in Chapter 6.

▶ *Surgery* offers some people long-lasting symptom relief. Although the inflamed sections of the intestine are removed, it's not a cure. Crohn's disease tends to reappear near areas of removed intestine.

Doctors can soothe inflamed intestines with a one-two punch using prescription medications. Anti-inflammatories like these deliver the first punch when they ease inflammation.

Remicade, a drug given by injection, was approved as an effective treatment for Crohn's disease several years ago. Recently, it was also approved to treat ulcerative colitis. That's because both Crohn's and UC rev up the amount of tumor necrosis factor (TNF) your body naturally produces — a sure way to fire up inflammation. But Remicade helps limit the amount of TNF and short-circuits inflammation. Remicade isn't for everyone. Some people experience allergic reactions or stomach pain. Serious infections, including pneumonia and tuberculosis, are also possible. But this unique medicine may save the day when dangerous or intolerable side effects prevent you from using other drugs or when other drugs can't get the job done.

▶ *aminosalicylates,* like mesalamine

▶ *corticosteroids,* like prednisone or budesonide (Entocort EC). Exciting new research suggests that budesonide can help lengthen the time between symptom flare-ups.

Immunity regulators are the second punch. These drugs may prevent inflammation from happening in the first place.

▶ *immune suppressors,* like azathioprine (Imuran) and 6-mercaptopurine (Purinethol) or cyclosporine A (Sandimmune)

▶ *antibiotics,* like metronidazole and ciprofloxacin

▶ *Remicade* (infliximab), an FDA-approved drug that's a mix of proteins, antibodies, and genes from living organisms

▶ *Humira* (adalimumab), a drug usually prescribed for rheumatoid arthritis, could help if Remicade no longer works

Talk with your doctor before taking any drugs or discontinuing any medication.

Ulcerative colitis
Dealing with an inflamed colon

The average person may get diarrhea four times a year, but people with ulcerative colitis (UC) may experience it four times a day. If you are battling this exasperating disease, think like a military general to help get those numbers down. Learn everything you can about your adversary, so you'll know the best ways to fight back.

What is ulcerative colitis?

Ulcerative colitis is a chronic inflammatory bowel disease, or IBD for short. It usually affects the lining of the large intestine, or colon. The inflammation generally occurs in the rectum and sigmoid colon, the lower part of the colon, but it can affect the entire colon. Different kinds of IBDs may cause inflammation in either the small or large intestine.

Common symptoms and early warning signs

Your colon recognizes inflammation as a warning sign of trouble, so it frantically tries to get rid of whatever is causing problems.

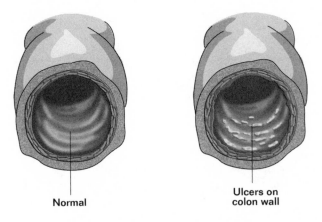

Normal

Ulcers on colon wall

Unfortunately, with ulcerative colitis, that can trigger symptoms like bloody diarrhea and abdominal pain. This inflammation also causes sores called ulcers. These can make your colon wall look ulcerated — cratered and battered like the moon. That's why it's called ulcerative colitis. But UC is called other names, too — names that describe how much of the colon gets inflamed.

▶ *pancolitis* — inflammation of the rectum, plus the entire colon

▶ *distal colitis, left-sided colitis, or limited colitis* — inflammation of the rectum, plus only the left side of the colon

▶ *proctitis or ulcerative proctitis* — inflammation of the rectum and anus, but not the colon

The good news about UC is that you may not experience symptoms all the time. In fact, your symptoms may flare up for awhile and then seem to almost disappear until the next flare-up. When you have symptoms, these are the most common:

▶ loosening of the stool

▶ bloody diarrhea

▶ weight loss

▶ rectal bleeding

▶ severe urgency to have a bowel movement

▶ abdominal pain

▶ fatigue

▶ loss of appetite

▶ loss of body fluids and nutrients

Some people might also experience poor appetite, fever, or painful rectal spasms. People with proctitis may experience constipation instead of diarrhea. You could also develop complications like these:

▶ arthritis

▶ liver disease

▶ skin rashes

▶ inflammation of the spine or pelvic joints

▶ inflammation of the eye

▶ osteoporosis

▶ anemia

▶ colon cancer

Are you at risk?

No one is certain what causes ulcerative colitis, but scientists suspect a faulty immune system could be involved. That's one of the reasons UC is tough to diagnose. Health professionals do know the disease tends to run in families and usually starts between the ages of 15 and 30 or, less frequently, between ages 50 and 70.

Medical procedures your doctor may order

Picking the right suspect from a lineup of digestive ills isn't easy. After a physical exam, your doctor might use these tests to help make a diagnosis.

Stool sample. A laboratory checks the stool sample you provide for either infection-causing microbes or for hidden blood that may be from bleeding in your colon.

Blood tests. Blood tests reveal signs of inflammation, like raised white blood cell count, below-normal levels of a protein called albumen, or something called an elevated erythrocyte sedimentation rate (ESR.) A low red blood cell count (anemia) might mean bleeding in your colon.

About 5 percent of people with ulcerative colitis develop colon cancer. The longer you have UC and the more of your colon affected, the more your cancer risk multiplies. If you've had UC for at least eight years, some experts recommend having a colonoscopy with biopsies every one to two years to screen for colon cancer.

X-rays of the abdomen. X-ray pictures may show signs of UC, like shortening of the colon or changes in its appearance.

Barium enema. After receiving an enema with barium, you have X-rays taken. Your doctor examines the X-rays for signs of UC, such as ulcers, shortening of the colon, or changes in its appearance.

Sigmoidoscopy or colonoscopy. Your doctor can use a long tube with a camera at the end to look inside your colon for inflammation, bleeding, and ulcers.

Biopsy. During colonoscopy or sigmoidoscopy, your doctor may take a tiny bit of tissue. This tissue can be analyzed to determine whether you have ulcerative colitis.

New research suggests that people who have ulcerative colitis have a higher risk of several other illnesses. These include asthma, bronchitis, arthritis, and psoriasis.

Enteroclysis or small bowel series. These tests use barium-enhanced X-rays to check the small intestine for signs of IBD. The small bowel series is part of the barium swallow so you just drink barium and have X-rays taken. The enteroclysis has more risk of side effects and injury but can reveal special kinds of intestinal damage. While you're under mild anesthesia, a thin tube is passed through your nose or mouth down to your small intestine. Barium, pumped through the tube, fills your small intestine before X-rays are taken.

Magnetic resonance imaging (MRI). An MRI can help determine the severity of your ulcerative colitis.

Computed tomography (CT) scan. This scan shows your colon wall, including any inflammation.

For more details about medical tests, see Chapter 7.

Nutritional defense against ulcerative colitis

Your intestine responds to what you eat and drink, so choose a diet that will help it heal. Here's how to start.

▶ **Pass up raw fruits and vegetables,** especially fruits that may have a laxative effect, like prunes, fresh cherries, and peaches.

▶ **Try psyllium fiber,** the active ingredient in Metamucil and Fiberall. Psyllium could improve conditions in your colon, according to one animal study. And a small study of UC sufferers in remission suggested that psyllium may ease bowel disturbances. In one study, psyllium seeds helped decrease flare-ups just as well as mesalamine — a prescription drug. What's more, doctors may recommend psyllium for diarrhea from ulcerative colitis as long as it isn't severe.

▶ **Be picky about fiber,** especially when your symptoms are active. In his book, *The Maker's Diet,* Jordan S. Rubin, a doctor of naturopathic medicine, warns against eating bran fiber, the insoluble fiber found in grains and cereals. Rubin recommends low-carbohydrate foods that are high in fiber, like berries, celery, and fruits and vegetables with edible skins. Other authorities caution that cruciferous vegetables, like broccoli and cauliflower, especially when eaten raw, may cause problems as bulky chunks of fiber may not pass easily through the ulcerated colon.

▶ **Cut back on greasy foods,** fried foods, and caffeine to help prevent diarrhea, cramping, and gas.

▶ **Avoid alcohol and red pepper.** If other spicy foods trigger symptoms, avoid them, too.

▶ **Eliminate milk and milk products** if you're lactose intolerant or think you might be. These are frequent triggers for symptoms of UC and other IBDs.

▶ **Stay away from high-fat food,** red meat, and processed meat to see if that relieves your symptoms or prevents a relapse.

For more information

Crohn's & Colitis Foundation of America, Inc.

386 Park Avenue South, 17th Floor

New York, NY 10016-8804

800-932-2423

www.ccfa.org

United Ostomy Association, Inc.

36 Executive Park, Suite 120

Irvine, CA 92714

800-826-0826

www.uoa.org

▸ **Drink plenty of fluids.** The diarrhea that accompanies flare-ups can leave you dehydrated and feeling weak. The Crohn's and Colitis Foundation of America recommends you set a water-drinking goal based on your weight. Every day, drink one ounce of water for every two pounds you weigh. That's 100 ounces (about 3 quarts) for a 200-pound person.

▸ **Eat foods rich in antioxidants,** like selenium, vitamin C, and vitamin E, whenever possible. They neutralize harmful free radicals. Some researchers think free radicals contribute to IBD or make it worse. Also, ask your doctor if you need to take nutritional supplements. A shortage of nutrients is common in people who have IBD.

Additional steps to take

You can make simple lifestyle changes that will improve your symptoms and let you enjoy life again.

▸ **Keep a record of what you eat** and track your symptoms. This will help you identify foods that cause trouble.

▸ **Eat five or six small meals** a day instead of three large ones.

▸ **Learn to manage** and reduce your stress.

▸ **Get regular screenings** for osteoporosis, anemia, colon cancer, or other conditions linked with UC.

▸ **Avoid taking NSAIDs,** like ibuprofen and aspirin, unless you take them to prevent serious conditions, like heart attack or stroke. Ask your doctor about painkillers that won't irritate your digestive system.

▸ **Check with your doctor** about using psyllium or bran to add bulk to your stool if you have constipation from proctitis instead of diarrhea.

▸ **Ask your doctor about fish oil.** Omega-3 fish oil has anti-inflammatory powers. One study used fish oil to help people with UC manage their symptoms with fewer drugs. Although corticosteroids can control ulcerative colitis inflammation, doctors are concerned about their many long-term side effects.

▸ **Consider trying probiotic supplements.** Good bacteria, called probiotics, may help treat inflammatory bowel disease, including ulcerative colitis and Crohn's disease. The probiotic supplement VSL#3, which includes four strains of *Lactobacillus*, three strains of *Bifidobacterium*, and one strain of *Streptococci*, provides 450 billion live bacteria in each 6-gram dose. In a study of 20 people with ulcerative colitis in remission, 15 remained in remission for one year while taking 3 grams of VSL#3 twice daily. Early studies also suggest this supplement may help relieve inflammation in a related condition called pouchitis. You can read more about probiotics in *Crohn's disease* in this chapter and *Probiotics* in Chapter 4.

▸ **Get the latest facts** about turmeric or curcumin supplements. Animal studies suggest curcumin, a phytochemical found in the spice turmeric, might fight intestinal inflammation.

▸ **Consider bromelain.** Some doctors report that bromelain, an enzyme from pineapple taken as a supplement, helped people suffering with mild ulcerative colitis by healing the inflamed mucous membranes lining their colons.

An exciting study from The Cleveland Clinic suggests a new supplement might ease ulcerative colitis symptoms and help you cut back on traditional therapies, like corticosteroid drugs, which can have long-term side effects. The nutritionally complete balanced supplement includes fish oil, soluble fibers like fructooligosaccharides, and antioxidants, like selenium and vitamins E and C. Proportions of the ingredients aren't currently available. The product is manufactured by Ross Products and Abbott Laboratories and is currently being evaluated for introduction to the public.

Medical treatment options

Nearly 70 percent of UC victims respond to nonsurgical treatments, reducing their symptoms so much that they're considered to be in good health.

Eventually, some ulcerative colitis sufferers, about 25 to 40 percent, have their colons removed for various reasons. Sometimes other treatments don't help or a crisis develops. Surgery to remove the colon and rectum is called proctocolectomy, and it's usually combined with one of these procedures.

The FDA has recently approved Remicade as a new drug for ulcerative colitis — one that may help you avoid surgery when other treatments fail. This drug, given by injection, is already used as an effective treatment for Crohn's disease, the other major inflammatory bowel disease. You can read more about Remicade in *Crohn's disease* in this chapter.

▸ *Ileostomy* is a surgery that creates a small opening near the beltline so waste can leave the body and pass into an easily emptied exterior pouch.

▸ *Ileoanal anastomosis* replaces the removed organs with a pouch so you can go to the bathroom like you normally would. With this surgery, future inflammation of the internal pouch (pouchitis) is possible.

Most health experts say surgery should be reserved for only the most serious cases of UC, which haven't responded to other therapies.

Doctors use anti-inflammatory drugs to ease inflammation and immune suppressors to help prevent inflammation from starting. Your doctor may also prescribe drugs to relieve pain, diarrhea, or infection. Ask your doctor about these options.

▸ *Heparin.* According to the National Institute of Diabetes and Digestive and Kidney Diseases, researchers are studying whether heparin, a blood thinner, can help control ulcerative colitis. In small trials, heparin was effective in people who did not respond to corticosteroids. Researchers think it interferes with the inflammation response but more research is needed.

▸ **Nicotine patch.** If you have ulcerative colitis and medication hasn't helped, ask your doctor about trying a nicotine patch. In one study, twice as many people with UC went into remission after six weeks using a nicotine patch as did people taking a placebo. However, the nicotine patch and nicotine gum are experimental and controversial. You can buy them without a prescription, but talk with your doctor first. The nicotine patch can cause side effects, and some people shouldn't use it. For more information, see *Nicotine patch* in Chapter 6.

Talk with your doctor before taking any drugs or discontinuing any medication.

Colon cancer
Early warning saves lives

Approximately 75 percent of the 150,000 people diagnosed with colon cancer in the United States each year don't have colon cancer in their family's history. But the good news is you can help dodge this deadly disease by taking the right steps — right now.

What is colon cancer?

You may not know it, but your colon and rectum constantly cast off old cells and add new ones. Your body usually does a super job of replacing old or dying cells with just the right number and kind of new cells. But sometimes the orderly growth of cells gets out of control. You may get cells that grow too fast, cells that grow in the wrong place, or too many new cells. When this happens, the cluster of extra cells is called a tumor. If the tumor is made of normal cells, it's called

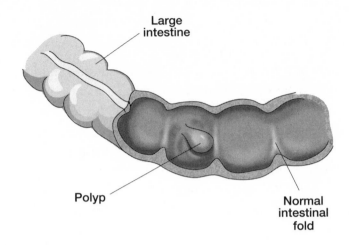

Large intestine

Polyp

Normal intestinal fold

a benign tumor. When cancer cells form the tumor, you will hear it called a malignant tumor.

Almost all colon cancer begins as polyps, which are at first benign tumors. In the early stages, they are usually small and produce few symptoms. If your doctor removes them, they probably won't cause further problems. If they're allowed to grow, some types of polyps may become cancerous.

If caught early, colon cancer is curable in about 90 percent of the people who develop it, but that number drops to 40 percent once the cancer spreads to lymph nodes or other organs.

Common symptoms and early warning signs

Colon cancer symptoms can be vague and easy to mistake for other problems, like constipation and hemorrhoids, or you may not have any symptoms at all. Keep an eye out for problems like these.

- ▶ unexplained weight loss
- ▶ black or tarry stools
- ▶ abdominal pain, possibly with cramps

- bleeding from your rectum

- a feeling of pressure in your rectum

- thin ribbon-like or rope-like stools

- morning diarrhea

- blood or mucus in the stools

- a feeling of pressure as if you still need to go to the bathroom after you're done

- fatigue and weakness

- alternating constipation and diarrhea

- persistent diarrhea

Are you at risk?

You are more likely to get polyps and colon cancer if you have these risk factors:

- **Family history.** Someone in your family has had polyps or colon cancer. Your risk goes up if the person is a close relative, if cancer occurred before age 45, or if several of your relatives have been diagnosed with colon cancer or precancerous polyps.

- **Age.** You are older than 50.

- **Inflammatory bowel disease.** You have ulcerative colitis or Crohn's disease.

- **Unhealthy lifestyle.** You eat a lot of fatty foods, smoke, drink alcohol, don't exercise, or are overweight.

Medical procedures your doctor may order

These tests help find hidden colon cancer early, giving you a better chance of beating the disease.

Colonoscopy. Your doctor uses a long, thin tube tipped with a tiny camera to see your colon from the inside. He looks for

The truth about other digestive cancers

Colon cancer is the second most common cancer in the United States and Europe, but these less-common digestive cancers are deadlier.

Esophageal cancer. At least 90 percent of the people diagnosed with cancer of the esophagus will die within five years. More than 13,000 deaths occurred in 2004 and 14,000 new cases were diagnosed, according to National Cancer Institute (NCI) estimates. Risk factors include being overweight, heavy smoking, heavy or chronic alcohol use, being male, having either GERD or Barrett's esophagus, being between 50 and 70 years old, and eating a diet low in fresh fruits and vegetables or high in nitrosamines (chemical compounds formed from nitrites in cured meats, beer, and other foods).

Stomach cancer. The NCI estimates this cancer, also called gastric cancer, caused over 11,000 deaths in 2004 and more than 22,000 new cases were diagnosed. Nearly 90 percent of the victims die within five years of diagnosis. *H. pylori* infection is the number one cause of stomach cancer, according to Barry Marshall, M.D., who won the Nobel Prize for his work. Other risk factors include tobacco use; high alcohol use; a diet high in salted, pickled or smoked foods; a family history of stomach cancer; deficiencies of vitamins A, C, or E; a diet low in selenium, beta carotene, or fiber; and being male or over age 50.

Pancreatic cancer. More than 95 percent of the people diagnosed with pancreatic cancer die within five years — the majority within a year. Around 31,800 new cases were diagnosed in 2004 and over 31,200 of these people died, the NCI estimates. Risk factors include smoking, a family history of pancreatic cancer, chronic alcohol abuse, a diet high in fat or meat, chronic pancreatitis, diabetes, and being between ages 60 and 70.

Liver cancer. NCI estimates say that 18,000 cases of liver cancer were diagnosed in 2004, causing over 14,000 deaths. Around 94 percent of the victims die within five years of diagnosis. Risk factors include high alcohol use, a family history of liver cancer, cirrhosis of the liver, exposure to hepatitis B virus or hepatitis C virus, and being male or over age 55.

polyps and damaged areas that could become cancerous. Instruments passed through the tube can remove a polyp or take a small tissue sample called a biopsy. Mild anesthesia and painkillers can help make this test more comfortable for you.

Flexible sigmoidoscopy. Your doctor uses a long, thin tube with a camera attached to examine the last third of your colon from the inside. He hunts for cancer, polyps, and damaged areas that could become cancerous.

Fecal occult blood test. You provide a stool sample, and the lab checks it for hidden blood. Some polyps and cancer reveal themselves by bleeding.

Digital rectal exam. Your doctor checks for tumors inside your rectum with a gloved finger.

Double contrast barium enema. For extra detail on X-rays, air is blown into your colon, and you're given an enema with barium, a contrast dye. The X-rays taken can show small areas of cancer or potential cancer.

The American Cancer Society says less than half of all Americans over age 50 undergo colon cancer screening. If everyone were tested, thousands of lives could be saved each year.

For more details about medical tests, see Chapter 7.

Nutritional defense against colon cancer

Look at what you're eating and make these healthy changes to protect yourself from this life-threatening disease.

▶ *Get more fiber in your diet.* The National Institutes of Health says you're less likely to develop colon cancer if you eat a high-fiber, low-fat diet. That means load up on foods rich in fiber, like barley, bulgur, beans, and whole-wheat flour. Experts believe fiber grabs on to potential cancers in your digestive system and carries them out of your body with waste material. Fiber also encourages a process in your lower intestine that gets rid of certain bile acids that promote the growth of polyps.

▶ *Eat plenty of fruits and vegetables.* Get five or more servings a day of antioxidant-rich deep green, dark yellow, or orange fruits and vegetables for natural cancer protection. Good choices include citrus fruits, cantaloupe, mango, spinach, cabbage, broccoli, sweet potatoes, and squash.

▶ *Go easy on red meat.* European researchers found that eating red meat, and processed meat in particular, can increase your risk of colon cancer. Replace at least some of that meat with baked chicken or broiled fish.

In addition, avoid sugar, white flour, and other highly processed starches. In one study, women who ate the most of these carbohydrates increased their risk of colon cancer almost seven times over women who ate the least.

Additional steps to take

Regular screening is your best defense, but a few simple adjustments to your lifestyle might help reduce your chances of developing colon cancer.

▶ *Maintain a healthy body weight.* Researchers at the Centers for Disease Control and Prevention found an unmistakable link between obesity and colon cancer.

▶ *Stay physically active.* Thirty minutes a day of exercise could lower your colon cancer risk by a whopping 83 percent.

▶ *Stop smoking and limit alcohol use.* A recent study found smokers were more likely to have colon polyps than nonsmokers, and their polyps tended to be more aggressive.

▶ *Ask your doctor about aspirin therapy.* As part of the ongoing Nurses' Health Study, researchers found that women who took more than 14 regular adult aspirin each week cut their risk of developing potentially cancerous polyps in half. They also say people at high risk may find they have fewer and smaller polyps with this kind of aspirin therapy. Although this is good news, aspirin is not recommended for people with only average risk factors because of potential side effects. Check with your doctor first, but if you can tolerate at least two aspirin tablets a week, you might lower your risk by 25 percent.

▸ **Get extra calcium.** Researchers believe calcium may bind to bile acids and ionized fatty acids, keeping them from irritating your colon lining. Surprisingly, supplements of 700 to 1,000 milligrams a day seem to work better than calcium from food.

If colon cancer runs in your family, supplements of other vitamins and minerals, like folate and vitamin E may help keep you from getting this deadly disease. For example, people who took vitamin E supplements over a 10-year period had a 57-percent lower risk of developing colon cancer. Never take large doses of supplements without talking with your doctor first.

For more information

American Cancer Society
800-ACS-2345
www.cancer.org

National Cancer Institute
800-4-CANCER
www.cancer.gov

Medical treatment options

Surgery is the primary treatment for colon cancer. It can be as simple as clipping off a polyp during a colonoscopy. But your doctor may have to remove large sections of your colon if the cancer has spread. Chemotherapy and radiation are other standard treatments. These drugs are also used.

▸ **Bevacizumab (Avastin),** one of the newest drug treatments, may literally starve malignant tumors to death by cutting off their blood supply. Ask your doctor if this drug is right for you.

▸ **Vaccines** may help the immune system recognize cancer cells and kill them off.

▶ **"Designer" viruses.** Inherited genes can cause colon and rectal cells to become cancerous. New gene therapies hope to correct these DNA problems using "designer" viruses.

▶ **Celecoxib,** an NSAID (nonsteroidal anti-inflammatory drug) sold as Celebrex, is FDA-approved for reducing polyp formation in certain people, but there are serious concerns about its effect on your heart.

Talk with your doctor before taking any drugs or discontinuing any medication.

Gastroenteritis
Fend off foodborne illnesses

You've just finished eating a great meal at your favorite restaurant. You invite your dinner companions back to your home for an enjoyable evening. Just as the conversation starts flowing, you double over in pain.

What is gastroenteritis?

Stomach flu, food poisoning, traveler's diarrhea — all common names for gastroenteritis, an infection that attacks your digestive tract. Many culprits cause it, including viruses, bacteria, and parasites.

Once inside, these microbes set up house in your digestive tract, attaching to the cells along your intestinal walls and multiplying. You may start to feel symptoms within a few hours or days, depending on the kind of organism and how many made it into your digestive system. These three illnesses are the most common forms of gastroenteritis — food poisoning, stomach flu, and traveler's diarrhea.

Most people get gastroenteritis from eating contaminated food — usually food that wasn't prepared properly, cooked thoroughly, or refrigerated quickly enough, or drinking water in places with poor water treatment.

The bacteria behind food poisoning are everywhere, but they're most abundant in meat, poultry, eggs, and milk. These bacteria produce a toxin that causes your intestines to secrete salt and water. The bowel becomes overwhelmed with fluid, causing diarrhea.

Viral gastroenteritis is commonly called stomach flu, but it's not caused by the influenza virus that attacks your respiratory system. These viruses invade the wall of your small intestine, damaging it so it leaks water and nutrients. As a result, you end up with watery stool. Symptoms usually improve in one to three days, but they can last as long as 10 days.

Several viruses cause viral gastroenteritis, including the rotavirus, astrovirus, and Norwalk and Sapporo viruses. All are highly contagious. They are often passed from person to person via unwashed hands; by sharing food, drink, utensils, or even towels with an infected person; or from eating food like undercooked oysters harvested in contaminated waters.

You can find foods from all over the world at your grocery store. Some foods were once only available seasonally. Now, foods from less-reliable foreign sources are found in stores year round. This contributes to the threat of food poisoning.

Aptly named, traveler's diarrhea usually strikes people traveling in developing countries with poor water treatment systems. Some of the same organisms behind food poisoning and stomach flu also cause traveler's diarrhea. The usual culprits are the bacterium *E. coli* and the Norwalk virus.

Here's a snapshot of the organisms that commonly cause gastroenteritis and how you are most likely to catch them.

Common causes of gastroenteritis	
Organism	**Source**
Campylobacter jejuni	contaminated water, raw milk, and raw or undercooked meat, poultry, or shellfish
Clostridium botulinum	improperly canned foods, garlic in oil, vacuum-packed and tightly wrapped food
Clostridium perfringens	foods left for long periods in steam tables or at room temperature
Escherichia (E.) coli	contaminated water, raw milk, raw or rare ground beef, unpasteurized apple juice or cider, uncooked fruits and vegetables
Listeria monocytogenes	soft cheese, raw milk, improperly processed ice cream, raw leafy vegetables, meat, and poultry
Salmonella	seafood, raw milk and dairy products, raw or undercooked eggs, poultry, and meat
Shigella	food, especially salads, prepared and handled by workers with poor personal hygiene
Staphylococcus aureus	transmitted from people to food through improper food handling, multiplies rapidly at room temperature, even heat won't kill this bacterium's toxins
Vibrio parahemolyticus	raw and undercooked shellfish
Entamoeba histolytica	contaminated food or water
Rotavirus	unwashed hands of people who have the virus; sharing food, drink, or utensils with people who have the virus
Norwalk virus	person to person contact, contaminated food or water, usually raw or undercooked oysters harvested in contaminated water
Astrovirus	unwashed hands of people who have the virus; sharing food, drink, or utensils with people who have the virus
Giardia	contaminated water, person-to-person contact
Cryptosporidium	contaminated water, person-to-person contact

Common symptoms and early warning signs

These symptoms of gastroenteritis can show up within hours of exposure or several days later.

- mild to severe diarrhea, sometimes bloody
- loss of appetite
- nausea or vomiting
- cramps and abdominal pain
- fever, muscle aches, or chills
- intestinal rumbling, especially in traveler's diarrhea

Most people recover from gastroenteritis in a matter of days, but see your doctor if you:

- go more than 24 hours without being able to keep down liquids.
- vomit for more than two days.
- have diarrhea for more than three days.
- notice blood in your vomit or stool.
- experience signs of dehydration, such as dizziness, dry mouth, excessive thirst, dark-yellow urine, or little or no urine.
- have a fever higher than 101 degrees Fahrenheit.

Are you at risk?

In general, people with weakened immune systems face the greatest threat from gastroenteritis. Older adults fall into that category, particularly those in nursing homes, because the immune system works less well with age. So do children under the age of six because their immune system is not fully formed yet.

People with liver disease are especially vulnerable to food poisoning caused by the *Vibrio vulnificus* bacterium sometimes found in raw and undercooked oysters.

Medical procedures your doctor may order

Determining if you have food poisoning, traveler's diarrhea, or stomach flu usually involves answering your doctor's questions about how you're feeling, when you first felt sick, what you've eaten lately,

Slash your risk of hepatitis A

The highly contagious hepatitis A virus leads to liver inflammation. It's a foodborne illness spread mostly through contaminated food and water.

Most people with hepatitis A have no obvious symptoms. However, older adults may have more severe symptoms, including these:

- nausea
- loss of appetite
- diarrhea
- dark urine or light-colored stools
- jaundice, or yellowing of the eyes and skin

- fatigue
- abdominal pain
- headaches
- easy bruising
- fever

Some people are in more danger of catching this disease than others. Day-care workers, children in day-care centers, people who live with someone infected with hepatitis A, and those who travel to countries where the illness is common are most likely to get it. Yet, you can slash your risk several easy ways.

- Wash your hands after using the bathroom and before handling food.
- Wear gloves if you have to handle someone's stool, and wash your hands afterward.
- Drink bottled water when you are in another country.
- Don't use ice cubes made from tap water in developing countries or wash food in it.

Your doctor can order a blood test to check for hepatitis A. Most cases heal on their own within six months, usually without damaging the liver.

and if anyone else you've eaten with recently has similar symptoms. Your doctor may also order one or more of the following tests to help find out what's causing your symptoms.

Stool test. You provide a sample or the doctor may take a rectal swab. A laboratory checks the sample for bacteria or parasites.

Blood test. A laboratory checks a sample of your blood for bacteria or parasites that cause food poisoning.

Food test. If a sample of a suspected food is available, it might be tested, too. If your doctor thinks food poisoning is behind your misery, this may help identify specifically which type of food poisoning you have.

Urine test. You "fill the cup" and a laboratory checks for microbes that cause food poisoning.

Sigmoidoscopy. This is used when your doctor thinks other illnesses, like ulcerative colitis, might be causing your symptoms. Your doctor uses a long, thin tube with a camera attached to examine the lower third of your colon.

For more details about medical tests, see Chapter 7.

Nutritional defense against gastroenteritis

Your digestive system needs some tender, loving care when you have gastroenteritis. These simple tips will help you feel better faster.

▶ **Drink as much fluid as possible throughout the day.** Take small, frequent sips if you are vomiting. Stay away from carbonated drinks, teas, sports drinks, caffeinated beverages, and fruit juices if you suspect you have gastroenteritis. Extreme diarrhea can cause fatal dehydration within 24 hours. Replacing lost fluids and electrolytes (salts) is crucial. Your best bet is to drink rehydrating solutions, such as Pedialyte, Oralyte, or Rehydralyte. Don't rely on sports drinks, such as Gatorade, which have relatively low amounts of electrolytes, to replace lost fluids if you have diarrhea.

▸ **Add bland foods slowly as your symptoms subside.** The BRAT diet — bananas, rice, applesauce, and toast — is a good option. Other easily digestible foods include gelatin, crackers, and cooked cereals.

▸ **Avoid dairy products for several days,** as well as caffeine, alcohol, fatty or spicy foods, and aspirin and other nonsteroidal anti-inflammatory drugs (NSAIDs).

Additional steps to take

Prevention truly is the best medicine. Be on the lookout for risky foods and hygiene hazards, and try these tips to protect yourself from harmful bacteria and viruses.

▸ **Avoid cooking or serving food** to others if you have diarrhea. Some forms of gastroenteritis are highly contagious.

▸ **Clean surfaces** before preparing food on them.

▸ **Handle food properly.** Always wash your hands before touching food and after using the bathroom, changing diapers, or handling pets.

▸ **Discard any can of food that bulges.** It may contain a deadly toxin produced by *Clostridium botulinum* bacteria in oxygen-restricted environments.

▸ **Use your refrigerator,** cold running water, or your microwave to defrost food — not your kitchen counter.

▸ **Marinate food** in your refrigerator.

▸ **Prevent cross-contamination.** Bacteria spreads from one food to another and can get on cutting boards, knives, and countertops. Wash your hands, utensils, and cutting boards between foods, especially after they come in contact with raw meat, poultry, fish, shellfish, or eggs.

▸ **Cook food to the appropriate temperature.** Food, particularly meat, poultry, and eggs, must be cooked long and hot enough to kill harmful organisms. Cook eggs until the yolk is firm, and cook ground beef until it reaches an internal temperature of 160 degrees Fahrenheit. Use a meat thermometer to check.

▶ **Keep raw meat, poultry, seafood,** and their juices away from foods that are ready to eat.

▶ **Rinse fresh fruit and vegetables** under running water to wash off visible dirt.

▶ **Throw away the outermost leaves** on a head of lettuce or cabbage.

▶ **Place cooked meat on a clean plate,** not on one that held raw meat.

▶ **Keep cold food cold** and hot food hot.

▶ **Serve safe spuds.** Foil-wrapped potatoes can spell danger. Bacteria breeds under the foil wrappers on baked potatoes, so keep them piping hot until they're served.

▶ **Remove turkey stuffing** immediately and refrigerate it in a separate container.

▶ **Refrigerate leftovers,** perishables, and prepared food right away. If left at room temperature for more than two hours, they might not be safe to eat.

▶ **Divide leftovers into smaller,** serving-size portions for refrigerating or freezing to cool them faster.

▶ **Leave room in your refrigerator** for cool air to circulate.

▶ **Don't leave cut produce sitting out** at room temperature for longer than a few hours.

▶ **Reheat cooked food** to at least 165 degrees Fahrenheit.

▶ **Report your illness** to your local health department if you suspect something you ate or drank made you ill.

▶ **Drink only pasteurized dairy products** and pasteurized apple juice or cider.

▶ **Wash your hands thoroughly and often,** including under your nails, especially after

An estimated 76 million cases of food poisoning occur in the United States each year.

having a bowel movement. Warn other people in your household to do the same.

Take special precautions when traveling abroad, especially if you venture to developing countries. These tips can help keep you safe.

▸ **Don't buy food or beverages** from street vendors in foreign countries.

▸ **Drink only bottled or boiled water** or carbonated drinks in sealed bottles or cans. Check the seals when you buy them to make sure they have not been opened.

▸ **Avoid tap water** and ice cubes made from tap water.

▸ **Only eat thoroughly cooked foods,** and only eat meat, chicken, or shellfish that are hot when served.

▸ **Peel fruits and vegetables yourself,** and avoid raw fruits and vegetables that cannot be peeled.

▸ **Pack some chewable bismuth subsalicylate** (Pepto-Bismol) tablets when you travel. Experts say if you chew two tablets four times a day during your trip, you could avoid traveler's diarrhea.

▸ **Talk with your doctor** about taking the prescription antibiotic Rifaximin while traveling. New research shows it may prevent traveler's diarrhea caused by bacteria such as *E. coli*.

▸ **Carry small packets** of powdered rehydration solutions with you while traveling abroad. Look for packets of World Health Organization Oral Rehydration Solution. You can mix it with bottled water to prevent dehydration if you develop traveler's diarrhea.

▸ **Get more health tips** on traveling to specific countries from the Centers for Disease Control and Prevention. Visit their Web site at *www.cdc.gov.*

Prescription medications your doctor may order

Even though bacteria often cause gastroenteritis, some doctors may avoid prescribing antibiotics. That's because the drugs themselves can cause diarrhea, and health experts say over prescribing antibiotics can lead to drug-resistant strains of bacteria. Instead, your doctor is likely to advise lots of fluid and rest.

There are a few exceptions. If your doctor knows that Campylobacter, Shigella, or Vibrio bacteria are behind your illness, she may prescribe antibiotics.

Over-the-counter medicines made with bismuth subsalicylate, such as Pepto-Bismol, may ease diarrhea. But avoid taking any antidiarrheal medicine if you have a high fever or notice blood in your stool. They may make your illness worse.

Talk with your doctor before taking any drugs or discontinuing any medication.

Irritable bowel syndrome
Tame menacing flare-ups

First, the good news — irritable bowel syndrome, or IBS, is not a disease, and it doesn't harm your intestines. But that's small consolation for the millions of sufferers.

IBS can certainly make you irritable. Rushing to the bathroom, or the fear of having to rush to the bathroom, can interfere with work, travel, and social events. For some people, it can even be disabling.

What is IBS?

One in every five Americans has IBS. Of those, 80 percent are women.

Some doctors call IBS spastic colon or nervous colon because the nerves and muscles in the bowel are irritated or oversensitive. That makes your intestines either squeeze too hard or not hard enough, so your whole system works more slowly or more quickly than it should.

Unlike other gastrointestinal ailments, researchers can't point to a specific bacterium, virus, tumor, or immune problem as the cause of IBS, at least not yet, although some doctors think that a virus or bacterial infection may be one possible trigger for IBS. That doesn't mean it's a psychiatric problem or "all in your head." Scientists have shown that the colon of someone with IBS acts differently than a colon that is IBS-free. But they're still trying to find out why.

Key signs and symptoms doctors look for

If distressing symptoms are especially prevalent an hour or so after eating a meal, this may be suggestive of IBS. Or you have abdominal pain or discomfort for 12 out of the last 52 weeks, and the pain has one of these features.

▶ Going to the bathroom makes it go away.

▶ You have significantly more bowel movements after the pain starts, or far fewer than before.

▶ After the pain starts, your stools become noticeably harder or softer.

It's even more likely to be IBS if you also have one or more of these signs.

▶ You have more than three bowel movements a day or less than three a week.

▶ Your stools are either too loose or too hard in at least a quarter of your bowel movements.

▶ You need to strain when you go or you feel like you haven't finished after leaving the bathroom.

▶ When the urge to go to the bathroom hits, you need to go right away.

▶ You occasionally or frequently have abdominal bloating or swelling. Some people also have gas.

▶ You see mucus in your stool more than 25 percent of the time.

Meanwhile, health professionals do know that various factors, like stress and diet, may trigger or cause IBS symptoms. Fats are notorious for setting off symptoms, and many people discover that they're sensitive to other foods, too. Often, symptoms become worse during a woman's menstrual period.

Common symptoms and early warning signs

When you have IBS, you experience abdominal pain or discomfort along with constipation, diarrhea, or alternating constipation and diarrhea. Other symptoms include bloating, gas, cramping, mucus in your stool, and a feeling you have not finished a bowel movement. Fortunately, most people can control IBS symptoms by taking medication, reducing stress, and changing their diet.

Severe pain associated with IBS symptoms may indicate that a more serious, inflammatory condition, such as Crohn's disease, may be the cause of your problem. If severe pain is present, quick examination by a doctor is advisable to rule out appendicitis. Chronic pain with IBS symptoms may require evaluation by a competent gastroenterologist, a doctor specializing in the stomach, intestines, and related organs, to rule out Crohn's disease or other serious diseases.

For more information

International Foundation for Functional Gastrointestinal Disorders
P.O. Box 170864
Milwaukee, WI 53217
888-964-2001
www.iffgd.org

IBS Self-Help and Support Group
1440 Whalley Avenue #145
New Haven, CT 06515
www.ibsgroup.org

Are you at risk?

You're more likely to develop IBS if one or more of these describe you.

▸ You're in your 20s or 30s, the time when IBS usually begins.

▸ You're a woman.

▸ One or more of your relatives has had IBS.

▸ You have depression or anxiety.

Medical procedures your doctor may order

Symptoms are the key to diagnosing IBS, so your doctor's office visit may be the most important thing you can do. These tests can also help diagnose IBS.

Physical exam. The doctor asks for many details of your medical history and symptoms. In addition to a regular physical exam, you may be given a digital rectal exam and, if you're a woman, a pelvic exam.

Flexible sigmoidoscopy. The doctor inserts a long, thin tube with a camera attached, called a sigmoidoscope, to see inside the lower third of your colon. Air may also be pumped in to help the doctor see your colon better. The insertion of the sigmoidoscope or air entering the colon may cause bowel spasm in people with IBS.

To rule out other problems, such as diverticulitis or colon cancer, your doctor may order tests like the barium swallow, ultrasound, barium enema, colonoscopy, FOBT, urine tests, stool tests, or blood tests.

For more details about medical tests, see Chapter 7.

That sweet tooth may be torture to your bowels, even if you use sugar substitutes. Many people with IBS have trouble digesting fructose and sorbitol. Fructose occurs naturally in fruit, corn syrup, and honey. Sorbitol, found in certain berries and apples, is used as a sweetener in sugar-free candy and gum.

Researchers in Israel asked IBS sufferers to cut these sweeteners from their diets for one month. Irritable bowel symptoms dramatically decreased in 50 percent of those who did this.

Nutritional defense against IBS

Experts recommend a low-fat, high-fiber diet to manage IBS. But what source of fiber is best? Does your digestive system benefit more from savory breads and cereals or from scrumptious fruits and vegetables? The answer may surprise you.

Some doctors have told patients suffering from irritable bowel syndrome, or "spastic colon," to eat more bran. Now it turns out that the insoluble fiber in bran only makes IBS worse. The good news is that new research affirms the healing power of soluble fiber found in several other foods for IBS.

Use these guidelines to help you feel better and avoid symptoms.

▸ **Choose gentler sources of fiber,** like noncitrus fruits and cooked vegetables. Peaches, carrots, kidney beans, broccoli, raw cabbage, raw peas, oat bran, apples, flaxseed, and lima beans provide plenty of beneficial soluble fiber.

▸ **Give pectin a try.** This soluble fiber is probably the best product for slowing down the passage of food associated with the intermittent diarrhea of IBS. Applesauce is sometimes advised, but sorbitol found in apples may aggravate IBS. Liquid pectin may be just what's needed to reduce IBS symptoms without compounding the problem. Liquid pectin,

A new study suggests that a special antibiotic, called rifaximin, may help some people who have IBS. Rifaximin stays in the gut instead of being absorbed into the bloodstream. In the small study, funded by the makers of the drug, people with diarrhea symptoms who took rifaximin for 10 days showed twice as much improvement as those who took a placebo, and the positive effects lasted for 10 weeks. The researchers think the drug might kill an overpopulation of bacteria in the small intestine, a possible culprit behind IBS symptoms. Scientists hope to follow up with larger studies.

available in pouches, can be purchased in many supermarkets and drugstores.

▶ *Pour it on.* Drink plenty of water, at least six to eight glasses every day.

▶ *Avoid these foods* — chocolate, alcohol, soda, coffee, and fatty foods, like french fries, cheese, whole milk, and ice cream. Instead of coffee, drink herbal tea. You can soothe an irritable bowel just by sipping this beverage. Try peppermint, chamomile, or ginger for best results.

▶ *Take notes.* Keep a food journal to determine which foods trigger your IBS symptoms. Examples of wholesome foods that cause trouble for some people include wheat cereals, apples, and gassy vegetables, like broccoli and beans. You could also ask a registered dietitian for advice.

Additional steps to take

Living with IBS can be a challenge, but you can meet that challenge by making a few simple lifestyle changes.

▶ *Don't eat so fast.* You'll swallow less air if you slow down. Eat several small meals a day instead of three large ones. Or just eat less during each meal.

▶ *Get moving.* Researchers in Minnesota found that exercise can relieve IBS symptoms more effectively than changing your diet.

▶ *Chill out.* Find ways to manage your stress. Regular exercise, like walking, can help. So can relaxation techniques, like biofeedback, deep breathing, and aromatherapy. And make sure you're getting enough sleep.

▶ *Stay away from* caffeine, tobacco, and gum because these may aggravate IBS.

Remember to make any changes to your diet gradually to give your body time to adjust.

Medical treatment options

The Food and Drug Administration (FDA) has approved a drug specifically for women with severe IBS. The drug Alosetron hydrochloride, sold as Lotronex, helps women whose main symptom is severe diarrhea. However, the FDA temporarily withdrew this drug in 2000 because of serious side effects. It's available again but under strong restrictions.

Other remedies include antispasmodics, for help with diarrhea and pain, and antidepressants, for severe pain. Gentle laxatives, such as milk of magnesia, or fiber supplements can help relieve constipation associated with some cases of IBS. You'll want to avoid any drug whose side effects include stomach pain, nausea, diarrhea, or other digestive problems. Ask your doctor about these side effects whenever he prescribes a drug for you.

Talk with your doctor before taking any drugs or discontinuing any medication.

Lactose intolerance
Simple solution to stomach pain

You constantly have an upset stomach, but don't know why. The answer could be as simple as the glass of milk you drink every night before bedtime.

What is lactose intolerance?

Fifty million Americans are unable to digest lactose, the sugar found naturally in milk. These people are lactose intolerant — they don't have enough of an enzyme called lactase to break down the lactose in food.

Your body makes lactase in the lining of your small intestine. This enzyme breaks down big lactose sugars into smaller glucose and galactose sugars. Your liver then turns the galactose into glucose and sends it into your bloodstream to energize the cells of your body.

Common symptoms and early warning signs

After the age of two, you don't make as much lactase as when you were a baby, but you may not experience any symptoms. As you get older, your ability to digest lactose decreases even more.

This low level becomes a problem if you are lactose intolerant. When lactose enters your small intestine, it does not get broken down into smaller sugars. Instead, bacteria in your bowels feast on it, producing gas and other byproducts. This process leads to symptoms like these:

▶ nausea   ▶ abdominal cramps

▶ bloating   ▶ gas

▶ diarrhea

Lactose in common foods		
Food	**Serving size**	**Lactose content**
American cheese	1 oz.	1 gram
Butter	1 tablespoon	trace
Cottage cheese	1/2 cup	3 grams
Ice cream	1/2 cup	6 grams
Margarine	1 tablespoon	Trace
Milk, reduced-fat	1 cup	11 grams
Sherbet	1/2 cup	2 grams
Swiss cheese	1 oz.	1 gram
Yogurt, plain, low-fat	1 cup	5 grams

Some people who are lactose intolerant have an easier time digesting milk products than others. While some can handle small amounts of milk, yogurt, and cheese without symptoms, other people have to eliminate dairy altogether. Many health experts say most people who are lactose intolerant can digest one or two cups of milk a day, as long as the milk is consumed with meals.

Here's good news for people who can stomach small amounts of lactose — certain foods contain less lactose than others. That means you may still be able to enjoy them occasionally. Check the chart below for a quick comparison.

Are you at risk?

You are most likely to be lactose intolerant if you are of Asian-American, African-American, or American Indian descent, although this digestive disorder is not limited to any race or ethnic group. About 90 percent of Asian-Americans, 75 percent of African-Americans, and 75 percent of American Indians have this problem. People of northern European descent are least likely to be lactose intolerant.

Medical procedures your doctor may order

You can test yourself for lactose intolerance by cutting dairy from your diet for a few days to see if your symptoms go away. A doctor will confirm the diagnosis by asking you questions about your medical history and possibly ordering a lab test.

> *Discussing your self-test.* Tell your doctor if you've recently avoided dairy products for 10 days or more. Describe what happened to your symptoms. If you reintroduced a dairy item, tell when you did it, what the item was, and whether you had symptoms afterward.

> *Blood test.* A nurse takes three blood samples over the next two hours — after you drink some liquid lactose. If you're lactose

Read food and drug labels carefully. Lactose shows up in places you may not expect. For example, whey is the watery liquid that's left when milk becomes cheese. It, too, contains lactose and is a popular ingredient in many processed foods, like crackers. Also, keep in mind that 20 percent of prescription drugs and 6 percent of over-the-counter drugs contain lactose. Ask your pharmacist if you suspect one of your medications is a problem.

intolerant, your blood contains less glucose than most people would have after a dairy drink.

Breath test. After drinking liquid lactose, you exhale into a breath-testing device three times over a two-hour period. People who can't digest lactose have more hydrogen in their breath.

For more details about medical tests, see Chapter 7.

Nutritional defense against lactose intolerance

Who needs milk when you've got so many other options? The one good thing about this condition is you can stop the symptoms by simply giving up lactose, or cutting back.

▸ **Replace regular dairy products** with lactose-free products. Look for substitutes in health food stores or in the natural foods aisle at your grocery store. Rice milk, almond milk, and oat milk are all lactose-free, and they're often lower in fat and sodium than cow's milk.

▸ **Give yogurt a shot.** It's rich in calcium and lower in lactose than other dairy products, like milk and ice cream. Plus, the bacteria in yogurt actually help digest lactose.

▸ **Get calcium by eating** canned salmon with edible bones, raw broccoli, oranges, and pinto beans. Also, look for foods with added calcium. Fortified orange juice, for instance, has almost as much calcium as milk.

▸ **Focus on vitamin D.** If you've cut dairy from your diet, make sure to get enough vitamin D from other sources. Some cereals are enriched with this vitamin, so eating them with a milk substitute will cover your vitamin D quota without upsetting your stomach.

Additional steps to take

You don't have to make your own lactase enzyme — you can buy it as a supplement over-the-counter in liquid or tablet form.

▶ **Try adding liquid lactase to your milk** container and letting it sit for 24 hours. It will reduce the lactose in the milk so you can digest it more easily.

▶ **Take chewable lactase tablets** before lactose-laden meals or snacks so you can enjoy your food without a problem. Lactaid now makes a dietary supplement known as Fast Act that claims to work twice as fast as other products. Taken with the first bite of dairy, Fast Act may prevent symptoms, such as gas, bloating, and diarrhea, before they start.

▶ **Buy milk with added lactase,** such as Lactaid, NutriMil, and Parmalat, available at most grocery stores.

Celiac disease
Give gluten the heave-ho to soothe stomach pain

Man cannot live on bread alone, especially if he has celiac disease. This disease, often misdiagnosed as irritable bowel syndrome, can cause malnutrition, bloating — even cancer. Luckily, diet changes can reverse its symptoms.

What is celiac disease?

Celiac disease is a food intolerance to gluten, a protein in grains such as wheat, barley, rye, and oats. People with Celiac disease cannot digest this protein. When food with gluten reaches their small

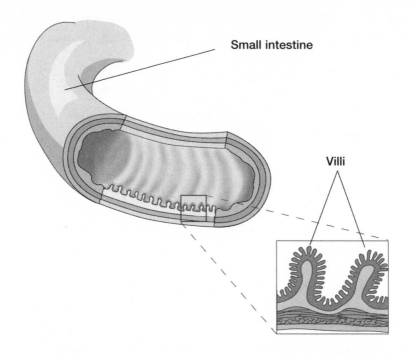

intestine, their immune system leaps into action, causing the intestinal wall to become inflamed.

Villi, tiny hair-like projections, absorb nutrients from food as it passes through the small intestine. But when the intestinal wall gets inflamed, the villi become irritated and damaged. Without enough healthy villi, you can actually become malnourished, even if you are eating nutritious meals.

Untreated, celiac disease can lead to osteoporosis thanks to poor nutrient absorption. The intestinal damage raises your risk of lymphoma and adenocarcinoma, two types of cancer. And a recent Danish study also found that people with celiac disease might be three times more likely to develop schizophrenia.

Common symptoms and early warning signs

Celiac disease remains largely underdiagnosed in the United States, but as much as 1 percent of the U.S. population may suffer from it.

Testing is rare, and people with the disease are often told they have irritable bowel syndrome or a nervous disorder. That's because symptoms are wide-ranging and variable. The condition usually develops in childhood, although some people do not see symptoms until adulthood. You might experience:

- fatigue
- weight loss
- bone, muscle, or joint pain
- diarrhea
- stools that float and have a strong, unpleasant odor

- abdominal pain
- stomach bloating
- irritability
- gas
- anemia

Or you may have no outward symptoms at all, if the undamaged part of your small intestine can compensate. But you still risk complications. These can include other conditions that may occur more frequently in those who have celiac disease, like liver disease; juvenile diabetes; thyroid disease; lupus; rheumatoid arthritis; Sjogren's syndrome, very dry eyes and mouth; and dermatitis herpetiformis, a burning, itching skin disease.

Are you at risk?

Also called celiac sprue, especially when it occurs in infants, celiac disease often runs in families, although it can be brought on by a viral infection early in life. This digestive disease affects about 1 in 300 people in Europe. Research indicates a similar, if not higher, occurrence in the United States.

Medical procedures your doctor may order

You may need special tests to get an accurate diagnosis.

Upper GI Endoscopy. A long, thin tube with a camera attached can help your doctor see areas of missing or damaged villi. You will be mildly sedated before your doctor inserts the camera-tipped tube into your mouth and down to your small intestine. The camera transmits images to a TV.

Biopsy. As part of upper GI endoscopy, biopsy of small intestine tissue will show damage to the villi.

Blood tests. Blood tests that check for antibodies called endomysial antibody or tissue transglutaminase antibody can

Get acquainted with tropical sprue

That recent vacation in the Caribbean, Central America, Southeast Asia, or southern India could have caused your digestive problems. People who visit, or live in, these areas are prone to tropical sprue, a disorder that causes an abnormal lining to develop in your small intestine.

This part of your digestive tract absorbs most of the nutrients you get from food. When the lining becomes damaged, it doesn't work as well. As a result, you could become malnourished and lose weight, even if you eat nutritious meals. Many experts think a bacterial infection may cause this rare illness, although they don't know for sure. Your doctor might suspect tropical sprue if you have recently visited a country where the disorder is common and you have several of these symptoms.

▶ chronic diarrhea

▶ light-colored stool

▶ unexplainable weight loss

▶ anemia

▶ sore tongue

▶ easy bruising

▶ prolonged bleeding after an injury

He may order X-rays of your small intestine, examine a stool sample, and take a biopsy — a small tissue sample — from your small intestine to look for signs of tropical sprue. If confirmed, your doctor may prescribe an antibiotic, such as tetracycline, along with folic acid and vitamin B12 supplements.

help your doctor determine whether to rule out celiac disease. The test called the gliadin antibody test is less accurate.

For more details about medical tests, see Chapter 7.

Nutritional defense against celiac disease

If you have celiac disease, an allergic reaction to gluten damages your small intestine. Cutting gluten out of your diet can repair this damage and help you live with the disease.

Unfortunately, that's easier said than done. Besides the obvious grain products, gluten hides in all sorts of foods, including creamed vegetables, salad dressings, gravies, sauces, nondairy creamers, herbal tea, and beer.

To beat celiac disease, you must strictly avoid grains, like wheat, rye, oats, barley, graham, wheat germ, durum, bulgur, triticale, spelt, and kamut. In addition:

> ▸ *Avoid malt or wheat starch,* which is often used to thicken sauces.

> ▸ *Fill up on plain meat,* fish, rice, fruits, and vegetables.

> ▸ *Eat breads and cereals made from* gluten-free flour, such as rice, corn, potato, amaranth, buckwheat, quinoa, millet, and bean flour.

Additional steps to take

Although it's a difficult, lifetime commitment, if you avoid gluten, you could see improvement almost immediately. Within three to six

For more information

Celiac Sprue Association
P.O. Box 31700
Omaha, NE 68131-0700
877-272-4272
www.csaceliacs.org

Celiac Disease Foundation
13251 Ventura Blvd., Suite 1
Studio City, CA 91604-1838
818-990-2354
www.celiac.org

Gluten Intolerance Group
15110 10th Ave. S.W., Suite A
Seattle, WA 98166
206-246-6652
www.gluten.net

months, your intestines could be back in working order. These suggestions will help you get started.

▸ **Read labels carefully** and ask questions in restaurants. If you're unsure about something, don't eat it.

▸ **Find a good dietitian** to help you make smart food choices.

▸ **Ask your doctor** about taking nutritional supplements. People with celiac disease often have trouble absorbing fat-soluble vitamins, like A, D, and K, and other nutrients.

▸ **Try bromelain supplements.** Bromelain, an enzyme from pineapple taken as a supplement, may help people with celiac disease digest food. Some health professionals think this might give the digestive system a chance to heal.

Gluten can pop up where you least expect it, even in communion wafers, which are made from wheat flour.

Diverticular disease
Keep your colon young with fiber

Most people think of diverticular disease as an unavoidable, natural part of aging, but it doesn't have to be. Learn to prevent diverticula from developing in the first place and protect yourself from dangerous complications.

What is diverticular disease?

When you strain from constipation, you put too much pressure on your intestines, which weakens the intestinal wall. Over time, the weak spots start to give, forming small pouches, or diverticula, in the wall.

Most of these pouches are small, ranging from one-tenth inch to 1 inch across. In rare cases, a diverticulum can get as large as six inches across. If you have diverticula, you have a condition called diverticulosis.

Diverticula are not usually dangerous. But undigested food and bacteria can get trapped inside the pouches and harden, causing the diverticula to become infected and inflamed. This condition, called diverticulitis, can lead to serious complications. Inflamed pouches may rupture, spreading infection into the abdominal cavity and nearby organs.

Once you have diverticula, they don't go away. Luckily, only about 10 percent of people with diverticulosis ever develop diverticulitis.

You may be able to prevent diverticula from getting infected or even forming in the first place by adding more fiber to your daily menu. Experts think diverticular disease results mainly from eating too little fiber and too much processed food. Foods rich in insoluble fiber,

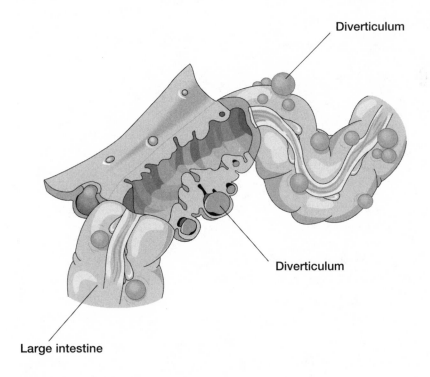

Diverticulum

Diverticulum

Large intestine

Why you shouldn't ignore abdominal pain — It might be appendicitis

The appendix is a small pouch attached to your colon in the lower right side of your abdomen. Although its purpose isn't known, it can cause big problems.

When the appendix opening gets blocked — by stool or swollen lymph nodes caused by a bacterial or viral infection — the whole organ becomes inflamed, a condition known as appendicitis. Once inflamed, it may rupture, a potentially life-threatening condition. Doctors can't save an inflamed appendix. They must surgically remove it.

Most people with appendicitis experience some of these symptoms:

▶ abdominal pain, first around the navel but later in the lower right abdomen

▶ loss of appetite

▶ constipation or diarrhea

▶ inability to pass gas

▶ nausea or vomiting

▶ abdominal swelling other symptoms develop

Generally, the abdominal pain gets worse when you move, take a deep breath, cough, or sneeze. You may also feel the urge to have a bowel movement to ease symptoms. If so, do not take laxatives or pain medication. Get to a doctor immediately.

Anyone can develop appendicitis, but most people get it between the ages of 10 and 30. Older adults, however, are more likely to suffer serious complications, because their symptoms are less noticeable. They may feel only mild abdominal pain and have no fever. Medical experts say if you are an older adult and experience a slight fever along with abdominal pain on your right side, call a doctor right away.

like whole grains, fruits, and vegetables, help keep you regular, bulking up and softening stool for easy passage through your intestines. No more straining during bowel movements could mean no diverticula forming.

Common symptoms and early warning signs

Diverticulosis does not usually cause symptoms. In some cases, however, people experience bloating, constipation, and pain in the lower left abdomen. But most often, you find out you have it by accident during an exam for something else. Diverticulitis can cause fever, chills, vomiting, diarrhea, constipation, loss of appetite, and pain in the lower left abdomen.

The pouches may bleed in both diverticulosis and diverticulitis, leaving blood in your stool. If you find blood in your stool, see your doctor. Usually the bleeding stops on its own, but if it persists, you might need medical treatment.

Are you at risk?

Your chances of getting diverticular disease go up as you get older. About half of people between the ages of 60 and 80 have diverticulosis, as does almost everyone over the age of 80. Luckily, the condition progresses to diverticulitis in only 10 to 25 percent of people.

This condition is very common in industrialized countries where people eat little fiber and lots of refined foods. In fact, the United States, Europe, and Australia have the highest rates of diverticular disease. But it's rare in developing nations, such as rural Africa and Asia, where people eat vegetable-rich, high-fiber diets.

Medical procedures your doctor may order

If your doctor suspects diverticular disease is behind your symptoms, he may suggest you have one or more of these tests.

Digital rectal exam. Your doctor checks for tenderness, blockage, or blood inside your rectum with a gloved finger.

Barium enema. You're given an enema with barium to help diverticula show up on X-rays. This test is not safe if your doctor suspects acute diverticulitis or if you have severe midsection pain.

Colonoscopy. Your doctor uses a long, thin tube with a tiny camera attached to check your colon for diverticula. Instruments passed through the tube can remove a polyp or take a small tissue sample called a biopsy. Expect this test if rectal bleeding is one of your symptoms. Although mild anesthesia and painkillers make this test easier, colonoscopy is not recommended if your doctor suspects acute diverticulitis.

CT scan. This detailed scan can check for diverticula when severe midsection pain makes a colonoscopy or barium enema unsafe.

Angiography. After giving you a sedative, painkiller, and local anesthesia, your doctor makes a small incision and inserts a thin catheter into a major artery near your midsection. X-ray pictures of the artery, called angiograms, are taken to pinpoint the source of bleeding.

Ultrasound. As a handheld ultrasound "scanner" is drawn over your midsection, a sonar-like device builds images of your colon with sound waves. Diverticula can show up in these images.

For more details about medical tests, see Chapter 7.

Nutritional defense against diverticular disease

Slash your risk of diverticular disease by eating more fruits, vegetables, and whole grains, like bran cereals and whole-wheat bread. This will relieve constipation and take pressure off your colon. A high-fiber diet will also ease symptoms for people who already have diverticular disease.

▸ *Eat at least 20 to 35 grams of fiber* every day. You can reach that quota by eating a bowl of bran flakes for breakfast, a sandwich with whole-wheat bread and a pear for lunch, and lima beans with your dinner. Even if you already have diverticula, improving your diet will keep more from forming. For additional fiber, include apples, peaches, broccoli, cabbage, spinach, carrots, asparagus, squash, and kidney beans in your daily menu.

▸ *Drink plenty of water.* It's especially important to drink plenty of water when you add more fiber to your diet. If you don't, you could end up with a blockage in your intestines.

▸ *Avoid these things* if you have diverticulosis — nuts, popcorn hulls, and sunflower, sesame, pumpkin, and caraway seeds. The National Institute of Diabetes and Digestive and Kidney Diseases says these hard foods can get trapped in the pouches, causing an infection.

Additional steps to take

Since constipation associated with inadequate fiber in the diet seems to be the main culprit in diverticular disease, try these tips for healthier bowels.

▸ *Exercise regularly* to help keep the muscles in your intestine toned. A mild workout often stimulates bowel movements.

▸ *Avoid taking* stimulant laxatives. They are designed to make your bowels contract, which can further irritate your colon.

▸ *Learn to relax* and manage your stress. This might help relieve your symptoms.

Medical treatment options

Medical treatment isn't usually necessary with diverticulosis. Symptoms usually improve dramatically when adequate bran or other types of insoluble fiber are added to the diet. Symptoms usually improve dramatically when adequate bran or other types of insoluble fiber are added to the diet. The most you'll need is a mild pain medication, if anything, but without adequate dietary fiber, it may progress to diverticulitis.

Diverticulitis requires more care. You may be treated at home with bed rest, antibiotics, and a liquid diet. If your case is severe, your doctor may hospitalize you and place you on intravenous antibiotics. Most cases, about 80 percent, of severe diverticulitis can be successfully treated without surgery. But if conventional therapy can't kick the infection, or if you experience two or more attacks of diverticulitis, you might need surgery to remove the infected part of your colon.

Talk with your doctor before taking any drugs or discontinuing any medication.

Anal fissure
Heal the damage with a simple plan

An anal fissure is a small tear or cut in the lining of your anal canal, and it makes bowel movements painful. The good news is you can help it heal quickly and prevent it from happening again.

What causes anal fissure?

Constipation is often the villain behind an anal fissure, but it may also be triggered by diarrhea, surgery, colonoscopy, sigmoidoscopy, childbirth, or too much pressure in the anus. Anal fissures may also be caused by other health problems, such as Crohn's disease, ulcerative colitis, a tumor, or sexually transmitted diseases.

Common symptoms and early warning signs

You'll have at least one of these symptoms if you have an anal fissure.

▶ burning pain that starts during a bowel movement and may last up to several hours afterward

▶ bright red blood on the outside of stool or on toilet paper after wiping

▶ anal itching

Hemorrhoids can occur along with fissures and often have similar symptoms. But pain during a bowel movement means fissures are probably present. Talk with your doctor and get started on treatment if your symptoms last longer than six weeks. Delays or the wrong home treatment could allow the fissure to become chronic — and that may require drugs or surgery. But surgery should be a last resort because most anal fissures will heal with patience and a diet supplemented with smooth, soluble fiber, like psyllium.

Are you at risk?

You're more likely to develop an anal fissure if you are between the ages of 30 and 50. Frequent bouts of constipation may raise your risk as well.

Medical procedures your doctor may order

Your doctor can check for an anal fissure with these exams.

Physical exam. Your doctor uses a gloved finger to examine inside your rectum. This might be painful if you have a fissure.

Anoscopy. The doctor inserts an anoscope, a thin, plastic tube about 3 inches long, into the lower part of your rectum. He checks for fissures as the scope is slowly withdrawn. You could feel pain if you have an anal fissure.

For more details about medical tests, see Chapter 7.

Nutritional defense against anal fissure

What you eat and drink may do more than just ease your discomfort, you may also help the fissure heal and prevent new ones from developing. Here's how.

- ▶ *Rediscover fiber.* If constipation is part of your problem, fiber-rich foods can help. Consider fruits high in soluble fiber, like peaches, apples, or apricots, to help soften stool and ease the pain. Add high-fiber foods gradually so you don't trigger bloating or gas. Also, talk with your doctor about psyllium supplements. According to one study, 44 percent of people with anal fissures were cured within four to eight weeks after taking psyllium supplements.

- ▶ *Just add water.* Drink more fluids, especially if you're adding more fiber to your diet. You'll help prevent the gas and other side effects a fiber boost can cause.

- ▶ *Add more vitamin C.* This vitamin helps wounds heal. Eat more foods rich in vitamin C, like citrus fruits, strawberries, and sweet red peppers. And don't hesitate to take vitamin C supplements up to 500 to 1,000 milligrams a day.

Additional steps to take

Up to 90 percent of all anal fissures heal on their own with simple at-home treatments like these.

- ▶ *Use a stool softener* temporarily. This helps make bowel movements less painful.

- ▶ *Avoid straining* when you are having a bowel movement.

- ▶ *Skip the creams.* Topical steroid creams and anesthetics may do more harm than good.

- ▶ *Take a warm sitz bath.* A 10- to 15-minute bath after each bowel movement can help relieve your discomfort, but make sure the water is warm, not hot.

- ▶ *Ask your doctor* if glycerin suppositories could help relieve your discomfort.

▸ **Wipe gently.** Do not rub or scratch, especially if itching occurs. You could make things worse.

Medical treatment options

Any anal fissure that isn't beginning to heal after six weeks of adding sufficient soluble fiber to your diet is considered chronic and may not heal without medical help.

▸ **Ointments** containing nitrate help heal the fissure. You'll put a little on the fissure several times a day for up to eight weeks. Side effects can include headaches, in some cases severe.

▸ **Calcium channel blockers,** drugs used to treat high blood pressure, can also help heal fissures. Nifedipine (Procardia) has a success rate around 60 percent when used for eight weeks, but you may experience side effects, like headache or swelling in your feet and ankles.

▸ **Low-dose Botox shots** have an even higher success rate, but the injection can be painful. Side effects include bleeding, blood clots near the anus, fecal incontinence, and a dangerous bacterial blood infection.

If drugs and natural treatments fail, your doctor might suggest one of these surgical procedures.

▸ **Dilation or sphincterotomy** may help by preventing anal spasms. During anal dilation, the surgeon holds the anus open for four minutes, stretching it to permanently reduce spasms and intense anal pressure. Side effects include excessive gas and fecal incontinence. Sphincterotomy, or cutting muscles in the anal canal, has a higher success rate and is less likely to lead to loss of bowel control.

▸ **Anal advancement flap** is a procedure speeds healing by removing the edges of the fissure and covering the remaining injury with healthy tissue.

Talk with your doctor before taking any drugs or discontinuing any medication.

Anorectal fistula
Find the cause of embarrassing symptoms

Even kings aren't immune to fistulas. King Louis XIV, one of the grand old kings of France, had a fistula problem that was cured by surgery.

What is an anorectal fistula?

It's an abnormal opening in the anal skin and often forms when a gland in the anus becomes blocked or infected. The gland may become abscessed, swelling up with blood or pus, which needs to be drained. Sometimes the abscess becomes deep and turns into a tunnel leading out to the skin that may be offset from the opening of the anus. This is an anorectal fistula or "fistula."

Although infections can lead to fistulas, Crohn's disease may be the underlying trigger. Other possible causes include tuberculosis, cancer, and bacterial infections.

Common symptoms and early warning signs

If you have an abscess or fistula, you may experience symptoms like these.

- throbbing pain and possibly swelling near the site of the abscess or fistula
- irritation of skin around the anus
- drainage of pus from the anal opening or near it

Are you at risk?

You are more likely to get a fistula if you're between the ages of 30 and 50. You may also be at higher risk if you have Crohn's Disease.

Medical procedures your doctor may order

About half of the people who have an abscess will also develop a fistula. Here's how your doctor will find out if you're one of them.

Physical exam. Your doctor uses a gloved finger to check your anus and rectum for fistulas.

Anoscopy. The doctor inserts an anoscope, a thin, plastic tube about 3 inches long, into the lower part of your rectum and anus to find the main opening of the fistula. Anesthetic may be needed for this exam.

Sigmoidoscopy. A camera at the end of a long, thin tube can show your doctor the lower third of your colon. He orders this test to rule out other possible diseases.

For more details about medical tests, see Chapter 7.

Medical treatment options

Unless you have an inflammatory bowel disease, like Crohn's, anorectal fistulas usually are treated with surgery. Surgeons have developed a way to turn a fistula into a trench that will heal on its own. Another newer surgical technique allows the sealing of the fistula with a unique kind of adhesive.

Fistulas caused by Crohn's disease may respond to drugs like metronidazole (Flagyl,) azathioprine (Imuran), or infliximab (Remicade.) For more information about these drugs, see *Crohn's disease* on page 81.

Talk with your doctor before taking any drugs or discontinuing any medication.

Additional steps to take

Although anorectal fistulas usually have to be treated with surgery, you can help yourself during recovery.

▶ *Sitz baths.* Soaking the buttocks and anal area in warm water several times a day aids healing.

▶ *Stool softeners.* These can ease the strain on an already tender area.

▶ *Mini-pads.* You may need to wear a mini-pad or gauze pad until the drainage stops.

Hemorrhoids
Simple ways to ease the pain

Even though the discomfort of hemorrhoids has been around for more than 4,000 years, you might be able to find relief for yours in just a few weeks.

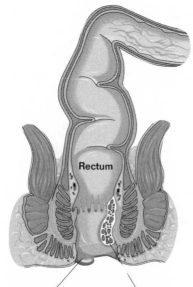

Rectum

External hemorrhoid

Internal hemorrhoid

What are hemorrhoids?

Hemorrhoids are a common medical condition. In fact, more than half of all Americans will develop hemorrhoids during their lifetimes, usually after age 30.

For many people, it's only a minor irritant that goes away quickly, but for others it means painful itching, swelling, and bleeding that affects daily living.

Hemorrhoids are veins around the anus that tend to stretch and swell under pressure, much like varicose veins in the legs. Veins inside the rectum cause internal hemorrhoids, and those just under the skin around the anus can cause external hemorrhoids.

Experts find it difficult to say that any one thing causes hemorrhoids, but there are several factors that can increase pressure on the veins located in your anus and rectum. The top cause of hemorrhoids in modern society appears to be a diet without adequate fiber associated with chronic constipation and the passage of hard, dry stools. Other causes may include:

- obesity
- straining, both on the toilet and when lifting or working
- chronic diarrhea
- sitting too long, either on the toilet or in a chair
- growing older
- liver disease
- prostate enlargement
- abdominal and pelvic tumors

If you have hemorrhoids, sitting or standing for a long time can make them worse.

Common symptoms and early warning signs

When external hemorrhoids are irritated, they cause pain and difficulty with hygiene. More pressure makes them bigger, often forming blood clots, and bleeding can start when they get scratched or break open. Mucous drainage and too much or too little cleaning can cause itching.

The only sign you may have of internal hemorrhoids is bright red blood on your toilet paper or in the toilet bowl. Sometimes these hemorrhoids push out through the anus and become protruding hemorrhoids similar to external hemorrhoids.

Are you at risk?

Half of all people over age 50 seek treatment for hemorrhoids. And check your family history. You can also inherit a tendency to develop hemorrhoids.

Medical procedures your doctor may order

To diagnose hemorrhoids, your doctor will ask you about changes in your bowel habits and other symptoms. Then he'll examine you for swollen blood vessels. He might also recommend these tests:

Outsmart mysterious, vanishing rectal pain

A sudden, excruciating pain in your rectum jolts you awake. It feels like a leg cramp — but in the wrong place. You get the urge to have a bowel movement, but nothing happens when you try. You may hurt so badly you sweat and go pale, but the pain vanishes in minutes.

If you've experienced these symptoms, you might have proctalgia fugax. It often occurs during sleep, while you're using the bathroom, or even during sex — but it isn't dangerous. You may have it a few times a year or several times a week. No one is sure why it happens, but some experts think proctalgia fugax might be linked with spasms from irritable bowel syndrome. Other health professionals point to food allergies.

In either case, popping an aspirin at the first sign of an attack can be effective but may not always help because the pain usually ends before the drug takes effect. To help prevent reoccurrence, try ice packs on the affected area followed by a warm sitz bath several times a day. See your doctor and ask him about the latest research and treatments.

Digital rectal exam. Your doctor uses a lubricated, gloved finger to check for hemorrhoids inside your rectum.

Anoscopy. This procedure uses a thin, lighted, plastic tube called an anoscope to examine inside your rectum.

Sigmoidoscopy or colonoscopy. Your doctor may order a colonoscopy or sigmoidoscopy to be sure that blood in your stool or toilet is coming from hemorrhoids and not from a more serious problem. Both tests are internal exams of the colon using a long tube with a camera. The colonoscopy examines more of the colon than a sigmoidoscopy.

For more details about medical tests, see Chapter 7.

Nutritional defense against hemorrhoids

Try these nutritional ways to relieve the discomfort of hemorrhoids.

▶ *Eat more high-fiber foods.* Fiber helps you avoid constipation, softens your stools so they are easier to pass, and relieves the pressure on your hemorrhoids. Try to get about 25 to 30 grams of fiber every day. Good sources include wheat bran, whole-grain foods, and fresh fruits and vegetables.

▶ *Try psyllium.* A 51-person double-blind study found that psyllium, a soluble fiber, reduced bleeding and pain in most people. Check with your doctor before trying psyllium supplements, like Metamucil.

▶ *Drink more fluids.* Six to eight glasses of liquid each day will help keep things moving. Stay away from alcohol because it draws water from your body and can cause constipation.

Additional steps to take

Simple lifestyle changes can help relieve your hemorrhoids, but if they don't go away in a week, see your doctor.

▶ *Take a footstool into the bathroom* with you and prop up your feet. This will prevent straining. If you don't have a stool, anything that raises your feet a few inches will help.

▶ *Rub a water-based lubricant,* like K-Y jelly, not petroleum jelly, around your anal area, inside and out, before having a bowel movement. This will help ease irritation. Preparation H may also be helpful, but some studies indicate it may be no more effective than other remedies.

Don't assume rectal bleeding is from hemorrhoids. Blood in your stool or on toilet paper is the most common symptom of hemorrhoids, but it might signal a more serious condition, like colon cancer. Blood can also come from a tear in your anal canal called an anal fissure. See your doctor to be sure. If an anal fissure is the diagnosis, think twice before having an operation to repair it. Surgery may be an unnecessary risk because the fissure usually will heal with a high-fiber diet and supplemental vitamin C to promote healing. A fissure that lasts longer than six weeks probably won't heal without medical help. Ask your doctor if you can try medication first.

▶ *Get up and move.* Moving around instead of sitting takes the pressure off the veins in your rectum.

▶ *Soak in a few inches of warm water* with your knees raised to ease the pain. Try three, 15-minute soaks a day.

▶ *Use an ice pack.* If your hemorrhoids are painfully swollen, take this as an excuse to rest. Stay in bed for a few hours with an ice pack on your anal area.

▶ *Help prevent constipation* by exercising regularly.

▶ *Maintain a healthy weight.* Being overweight is often a consequence of an inactive lifestyle and a poor diet.

Medical treatment options

If home remedies don't shrink your hemorrhoids, the doctor can choose more advanced medical solutions like these.

▶ *Rubber band ligation.* This inexpensive therapy is remarkably effective and much safer than surgery. A small rubber band, placed at the base of an internal hemorrhoid, cuts off circulation, and in about a week, the hemorrhoid withers and drops off.

▶ **Sclerotherapy.** Chemicals are injected into the hemorrhoid to make it shrink.

▶ **Laser heat or infrared light.** These destroy hemorrhoidal tissue.

▶ **Hemorrhoidectomy.** This surgical removal of internal or clotted external hemorrhoids is much riskier than other therapies. If your doctor recommends this surgery, get a second, unrelated opinion, because it's much riskier than other treatments.

Drugstore shelves are full of products for hemorrhoid relief. When you're trying to choose one, look for these ingredients.

▶ **Aloe vera gel** helps reduce irritation.

▶ **Hydrocortisone** relieves inflammation and itching.

▶ **Anesthetics** (benzocaine, pramoxine) can numb the pain.

▶ **Vasoconstrictors** (ephedrine, phenylephrine) reduce swelling and relieve itching.

▶ **Astringents** (witch hazel, zinc oxide) can help shrink swollen blood vessels.

▶ **Counterirritants** (camphor) work by soothing and comforting the irritated area.

Talk with your doctor before taking any drugs or discontinuing any medication.

Gallstones
Relief is a stone's throw away

A single stone can fell a giant. Anyone who has been hit with gallstones understands the painful truth of that statement. But there's good news — you may be able to manage your gallstones with a few simple diet and lifestyle changes.

What causes gallstones?

The story of gallstones starts with bile, a fluid made in the liver that helps digest fat. It is a combination of water, cholesterol, fat, salt, bilirubin, and protein. Bile travels from your liver to your gallbladder, where it stays until it's needed to help digest a meal. Once you have eaten, your gallbladder squeezes bile through tiny ducts, or tubes, and into your intestines to do its job.

The trouble usually begins when too much cholesterol, bile salts, or bilirubin builds up in the bile and stagnates in your gallbladder, where particles slowly form. These stones, as they're called, can be as small as a grain of sand or as large as a golf ball or egg. You can have

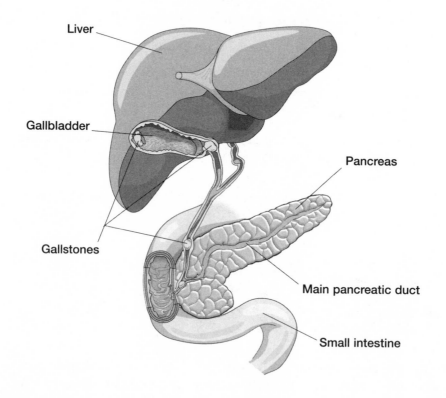

Liver

Gallbladder

Pancreas

Gallstones

Main pancreatic duct

Small intestine

a single gallstone or hundreds. The more stones you have or the larger they are, the more likely you are to have problems. Once they travel into the ducts and cause a blockage, those passageways become inflamed or infected, and you feel pain.

Common symptoms and early warning signs

Not everyone with gallstones has symptoms. Some people live a full life never knowing they have stones. But if a stone has blocked a duct, the pain is undeniable.

Gallstone pain can attack suddenly, often after a high-fat meal when your gallbladder is trying to release bile. You may hurt in your upper abdomen, but the pain can fan out to the area between your shoulder blades. You may also feel bloating, gas, indigestion, or even nausea.

Are you at risk?

Let your doctor know if you are at high risk for developing gallstones.

- ▶ *Family history.* Gallbladder problems may be in your genes. People of Norwegian, Chilean, or Hispanic descent, along with Mexican-American women and certain North American Indian tribes are much more likely to develop gallstones.

- ▶ *Age.* Your risk for gallstones rises after age 50, unless you remain physically active and maintain a healthy weight.

- ▶ *Gender.* Women are more likely to develop gallstones than men, especially young women. Hormones explain the difference, scientists say. The "gender gap" narrows with age, so older men and women have a similar risk of gallstones.

- ▶ *Medication.* A number of drugs increase your chance of developing gallstones, including ceftriaxone, clofibrate, estrogen replacement, progestogens, oral contraceptives, and octreotide.

- ▶ *Obesity.* Being obese may significantly raise your risk of gallstones, particularly for women. So does high cholesterol associated with being overweight. Obese people who carry their extra weight around their middle have the most risk.

Medical procedures your doctor may order

Most doctors use ultrasound since it's the most sensitive and specific test for gallstones. Other tests include:

Don't be tempted to ignore gallbladder problems. Stones can block bile flow if they lodge in the ducts that carry it from the liver to the small intestine. If ducts remain blocked for long, you can suffer severe damage or infection to your gallbladder, liver, or pancreas. Warning signs include fever, jaundice, and persistent pain.

CT scan. Your doctor may order a CT scan to figure out why you're having midsection pain. If gallstones are behind it, they'll show up on the scan. But a CT scan is too expensive to be ordered just for gallstones.

MRI. Magnetic Resonance Cholangiopancreatography or MRCP is a kind of MRI that's particularly good at finding blocked bile ducts.

HIDA scan. A HIDA scan follows the path of fats to either show blockages in the gallbladder, because the gallbladder doesn't fill up, or abnormal contractions of the gallbladder when it doesn't empty completely.

ERCP. This test uses a camera at the end of a long tube to find gallstones. Instruments passed through the tube can remove the stones.

Blood tests. A simple blood test can detect signs of blockage or infection. A higher-than-normal white blood cell count or something called an elevated erythrocyte sedimentation rate (ESR) may mean you have inflammation. The levels of several other substances in your blood, like bilirubin, might be outside the normal range if you have gallstones or gallbladder disease.

For more details about medical tests, see Chapter 7.

Nutritional defense against gallstones

Take steps to prevent gallstones in the first place, and you'll never have to suffer this painful condition. Here's how you can beat gallstones.

▸ *Favor fiber.* High levels of blood cholesterol increase your risk of having gallstones, but a high-fiber diet can help lower it. Here's why. Gallstones are generally absent in people who consume lots of dietary fiber. But in modern societies, when the diet is depleted of fiber, the body reabsorbs too much cholesterol, leading to not only heart disease but also gallstones that precipitate out of bile, which is supersaturated with cholesterol salts. Soluble fiber in the intestines absorbs bile that contains cholesterol salts and flushes them out of your body, while insoluble fiber helps move digestive products along. Adequate dietary fiber can help prevent gallstones. Try replacing sugars and fats with whole grains, fruits, and vegetables.

▸ *Avoid crash diets.* An astonishing percentage of painful gallstone attacks, especially in women, are preceded by rapid weight loss. Crash diets don't cause gallstones, but stones that have already formed in the gallbladder tend to move into the bile duct and cause painful spasms during ultra-low calorie diets.

▸ *Forsake fat.* Too much saturated fat slows digestion, makes your gallbladder work overtime, and elevates cholesterol, the chief ingredient in most gallstones.

▸ *Say no to sweets and sugar.* Sugar increases insulin production, which raises your cholesterol.

▸ *Keep drinking coffee.* Its caffeine might help. A study found that men who drank two or three cups a day were less likely to develop painful stones

Cholesterol is the main ingredient in most gallstones. Both fasting and crash dieting actually enrich the bile in your gallbladder with more cholesterol. What's more, medications aimed at reducing cholesterol do, too. These can increase your risk of a gallstone attack.

than abstainers. Another study found coffee relieved symptoms in women who already had gallstones.

▶ **Snack on nuts.** Women who ate the most peanuts and other nuts had a 25-percent lower risk of having their gallbladders surgically removed than women who never or rarely ate nuts, according to a recent Harvard study. It's possible the fatty acids in nuts, and other components, such as fiber, phytosterols, and magnesium, could contribute to the reduced risk of developing gallstones.

▶ **Change cholesterol with vitamin C.** Most gallstone sufferers are women, but researchers have found that women with high levels of vitamin C have less gallbladder disease. Vitamin C may protect by helping to convert cholesterol into bile acids.

Additional steps to take

Knowing your risk factors for gallstones can help you avoid this painful condition.

▶ **Take control of your weight.** Obesity is a major risk factor. Just remember — if you need to lose weight, do it gradually. Rapid weight loss causes the liver to secrete extra cholesterol into the bile.

▶ **Talk with your doctor about estrogen risk.** Scientists think estrogen may contribute to gallstones because it also increases the amount of cholesterol in your bile. Hormone replacement therapy and birth control pills are factors, so women are more likely than men to have gallstones.

Medical treatment options

People who have gallstones but no symptoms don't need medical treatment, experts say. Those who have recurring attacks, however, may decide to have their gallbladder removed, a procedure called cholecystectomy. Doctors nowadays do this using a laparoscope, which requires only several small incisions in your abdomen. In the hands of a skilled doctor, this procedure is much safer, much easier, and less painful than traditional surgery.

Doctors can also use ultrasonic shock waves to break up and dissolve stones, but many medical experts say this procedure is not very effective, and more stones usually develop.

People who cannot undergo surgery can have their gallbladder drained. Doctors make a small cut in the abdomen, slide a tube into the gallbladder, and drain it.

Some people can also get relief by having a small stent, or tube, placed in the gallbladder to keep it open. During this procedure, the surgeon can remove stones stuck in the ducts. Talk with your doctor about which procedure is right for you.

Pancreatitis
Best ways to keep your pancreas healthy

You may be surprised at how valuable your pancreas is, especially if pancreatitis keeps it from working properly. Although you may barely be aware of this gland nestled near your stomach and the top of your small intestine, your body depends on it for two important jobs.

▶ To produce the hormones insulin and glucagon. These hormones help regulate the glucose, a sugar, you get from food. Glucagon stimulates the liver to release glucose into your bloodstream. Insulin helps your body's cells use glucose, which gives you energy.

▶ To secrete digestive enzymes through the pancreatic duct and into the small intestine so they can help digest fats, proteins, and carbohydrates. The enzymes help your body convert food into fuel.

What is pancreatitis?

Pancreatitis means inflammation of the pancreas. Usually, pancreatic fluid contains digestive enzymes in an inactive form. As a safeguard, substances called inhibitors inactivate the enzymes that become active on their way to the small intestine. If a blockage occurs in the pancreas, the inactive enzymes overwhelm the inhibitors, and they become active and start to digest the pancreatic cells. This leads to pancreatitis.

Pancreatitis comes in two varieties. Acute pancreatitis (AP) happens suddenly. If severe, it can be fatal, but most people recover quickly. About 80,000 cases of AP occur in the United States yearly, and about 16,000 of those are severe. Up to 80 percent of hospital admissions for AP are due to either gallstones or alcohol. Heavy or long-term use of alcohol leads to clogs in very small pancreatic ducts, causing blockages.

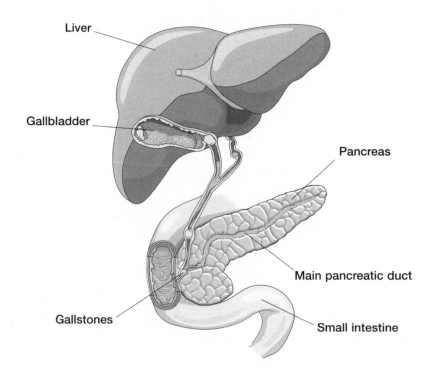

Gallstones, on the other hand, can cause a blockage in the major papilla — the last stage of the "drainage" system, which empties into the small intestine. Since the gallbladder and liver also use the major papilla for drainage, blockage by a gallstone can trigger pancreatitis by causing bile from the liver to back up into the pancreas.

Chronic pancreatitis (CP) doesn't go away and gradually damages, or even destroys, your pancreas. It can set in when inflammation is bad enough or persistent enough to damage your pancreas. This may happen after one or more "attacks" of acute pancreatitis.

Common symptoms and early warning signs

Stomach pain, usually in the upper abdomen, is frequently the first symptom of AP. But it takes different forms with different people. It may start out mild and get worse when you eat. Or maybe the pain begins suddenly and is severe or constant, and may seem to penetrate into your back. You may also see other AP symptoms like these:

▶ swollen and tender abdomen

▶ nausea or vomiting

▶ fever

▶ rapid pulse

To relieve pain from acute pancreatitis, remember this easy remedy. Sit up and lean forward. It might give you some relief.

Severe AP cases may lead to dehydration and low blood pressure. Pseudocysts, or buildups of fluid and tissue, are possible, as well as heart, kidney, or lung failure. If bleeding in the pancreas occurs, it can trigger shock and possibly death.

CP symptoms include nausea, vomiting, weight loss, and fatty stools. Most people with CP have abdominal pain, but others don't. If you have pain, it can resemble AP stomach pain. For example, it may get worse when you eat or drink or may penetrate to your back. In some cases, the pain goes away after awhile, probably because the pancreas stops making digestive enzymes.

People with chronic pancreatitis have a higher risk of pancreatic cancer. Ask your doctor about possible warning signs of this condition and whether he can recommend ways to lower your risk.

People with CP often lose weight, even though they still eat as much as usual. They can't absorb nutrients like they once did, because they no longer secrete enough pancreatic enzymes to break down food. Unabsorbed fats, proteins, and carbohydrates end up in the stool. If the pancreatic cells that produce insulin have been damaged, diabetes can develop, too.

Are you at risk?

Alcohol abuse is the leading cause of CP, but it is also associated with an increased inherited risk or can be caused by any of these:

▸ high levels of blood fats

▸ blocked or narrowed pancreatic duct due to pseudocysts

▸ congenital or autoimmune conditions

More men get acute pancreatitis than women, but in women, pancreatitis is more often a consequence of gallstones.

Medical procedures your doctor may order

You probably won't need all these tests to determine if you have pancreatitis. Your doctor will select the ones most likely to lead to an accurate diagnosis.

Medical exam. The doctor checks for an enlarged pancreas by pressing on your abdomen. He also asks about your alcohol use and medical history to see if you have signs of acute pancreatitis or its causes.

Blood tests. The pancreas creates the digestive enzymes, amylase and lipase. During acute pancreatitis, bloodstream levels of these enzymes are three times as high as normal.

Ultrasound of the abdomen. Like a sonar on a submarine, ultrasound forms pictures of your internal organs. If the images aren't dimmed by intestinal gas, your doctor checks these pictures for problems, like a swollen pancreas.

ERCP (endoscopic retrograde cholangiopancreatography). Using X-rays and a long, plastic tube tipped with a camera, your doctor examines your pancreas on a monitor. She might spot a narrowed duct, a gallstone, or something else that slows or blocks the exit of pancreatic enzymes. If needed, ERCP can be used to remove a stone.

X-ray of chest and/or abdomen. This may reveal problems like calculi (stones that indicate past inflammation) within the ducts, effects of pancreatitis on the lungs or intestines, or calcified gallstones that may cause a blockage.

For more information

American Gastroenterological Association
4930 Del Ray Avenue
Bethesda, MD 20814
301-654-2055
www.gastro.org

CT (computed tomography) scan. This scan can show the size and shape of the pancreas and may also uncover what's preventing pancreatic enzymes from leaving the pancreas.

Urine and stool samples. The bentiromide test works because people with chronic pancreatitis have low levels of a substance called para-aminobenzoic acid (PABA) in the urine. A special stool test can show whether you're having trouble absorbing fat, a possible sign of chronic pancreatitis.

For more details about medical tests, see Chapter 7.

Nutritional defense against pancreatitis

Dine wisely, and you may avoid painful trips to your doctor's office or the hospital. Get a head start with these tips.

▸ **Consider adding more vitamin C foods,** like citrus fruits, sweet red peppers, and cranberry juice cocktail, to your diet. Talk with your doctor about whether you should try vitamin C supplements. A recent small study from China suggests vitamin C may help protect against acute pancreatitis. What's more, extra vitamin C may help women avoid gallstones, which contribute to the problem.

▸ **Avoid fatty foods** if gallstones have caused your condition and your gallbladder has not been removed.

▸ **Cut back on foods high in refined sugars,** like desserts, pastries, and soft drinks, if you're worried about gallstones. Go easy on foods like pickles and cabbage, too.

Additional steps to take

Living a healthy lifestyle is one of the best ways to keep your pancreas in tip-top shape. These six steps will help you avoid pain in your pancreas.

▸ **Aim for a diet low in protein and fat** but high in carbohydrates.

▸ **Don't drink alcohol** or limit your consumption to no more than one 4-ounce glass of wine or 12-ounce bottle of beer a day. An equivalent amount (1 1/2-ounce shot) of alcohol in the form of distilled spirits will increase your blood alcohol level much more than when beer or wine is consumed. Alcohol contributes to blockages in your pancreas, which cause pancreatitis. Avoiding it may also help you have fewer and less severe attacks if you have chronic pancreatitis.

▸ **Avoid large meals,** especially right after an attack. To help prevent future problems, switch to four or five small meals a day.

▸ **Ask your doctor** whether you need supplements of the fat-soluble vitamins — A, D, E, and K.

▶ *Lower your triglycerides,* a type of fat that circulates in your blood. If high levels of triglycerides have led to pancreatitis, talk with your doctor about ways to lower them.

▶ *Stay up-to-date on new treatments.* An early animal study suggests rhubarb tablets from Chinese herbal medicine may help severe AP, but more research needs to be done. Talk with your doctor about the latest treatments.

Medical treatment options

For a mild case, doctors treat your symptoms until you recover naturally. But if your case is severe or caused by a blockage, you may need surgery, intravenous feeding, or another medical treatment. Chronic pancreatitis may necessitate surgery to unblock the pancreas or to remove part of it. You can sometimes avoid surgery if your doctor uses an endoscope — a long, narrow tube — to drain the pancreas.

Some medicines can irritate and inflame the pancreas. Fortunately, switching drugs can cure drug-induced pancreatitis.

Prescription medicines can be a double-edged sword. Some drugs help protect against pancreatitis, but others can actually trigger inflammation. Your doctor may prescribe medicines like these to help you feel better.

▶ *painkillers* for pancreatitis attacks

▶ *antibiotics* if an infection develops

▶ *pancreatic enzymes,* especially for chronic pancreatitis, when the pancreas no longer produces enough enzymes

Ask your doctor for his advice if you are taking any of these medicines. They may actually cause pancreatitis.

▸ *azathioprine* (Imuran) for rheumatoid arthritis and inflammatory bowel diseases (IBDs)

▸ *6-mercaptopurine* (Purinethol) for acute lymphatic leukemia and IBDs

▸ *trimethoprim-sulfamethoxazole* (Bactrim or Septra) for urinary tract infections or traveler's diarrhea

▸ *asparaginase* (Elspar) for acute lymphocytic leukemia

▸ *methyldopa* (Aldomet) for high blood pressure

Talk with your doctor before taking any drugs or discontinuing any medication.

CHAPTER 4

DON'T BE FOOLED BY THEIR MILD-MANNERED APPEARANCE. These secret weapons may look as unremarkable as Clark Kent, but

Best bets for better digestion

they can be every bit as powerful as Superman. They can help put an end to everything from minor heartburn and constipation to inflammatory bowel disease, ulcers, and even lower your colon cancer risk. Why not see for yourself? Jump-start your digestive health with these top seven best bets.

Fiber
Feast on whole foods to fight disease

Here's a diet plan to reduce constipation, varicose veins, and hemorrhoids. Simply eat more fiber. Your grandparents may have called it roughage, but this amazing substance actually helps your body run more smoothly.

Pioneering British surgeon Denis Burkitt uncovered this amazing health secret while working in Africa during the 1940s. He noticed that several diseases common in industrialized countries were rare in rural Africa. These included constipation, gallstones, hemorrhoids, diverticulosis, varicose veins, appendicitis, and hiatal hernias. The difference, he explained, was diet. People in developing nations tended to eat about 60 grams of fiber a day compared to the 20 grams or less eaten in Western countries. He realized that "dietary fiber," a term he coined, has remarkable properties that help the body avoid disease.

Healthy benefits

▸ Relieves diarrhea

▸ Calms IBS symptoms

▸ Softens stool

▸ Speeds stool through intestines

▸ Stabilizes blood sugar

▸ Eases pressure on hemorrhoids

▸ Fights colon polyps

▸ Helps prevent colon cancer

Fiber comes in two main varieties — soluble and insoluble. Soluble fiber, which dissolves in water, can be found in dried beans and peas, oats, barley, flaxseed, and many fruits and vegetables. You can find insoluble fiber, which does not dissolve in water, in whole-grain breads and cereals and fruits and veggies with rough, chewy textures. Your body can't break down insoluble fiber, but it does become mushy and moves without delay through your digestive system, keeping your bowels working smoothly and toning your digestive muscles. Many foods contain both soluble fiber and insoluble fiber, and both kinds offer many health benefits.

Read on to learn more about fiber, the secret "sponge" in your digestive tract that absorbs water and prevents constipation. You may be surprised at how many digestive conditions fiber can help prevent or improve.

Clobbers constipation. Fiber makes stool soft enough to cruise smoothly through your bowels. Water and other liquids help fiber keep things moving.

Eases heartburn. A recent study of 371 people found a link between eating a high-fiber, low-fat diet and a lower risk of heartburn or GERD symptoms.

Protects you from ulcers. Researchers discovered that fiber from fruits and vegetables could reduce your risk of ulcers. Fiber seems to encourage the growth of the protective mucous lining in your digestive tract.

Halts diarrhea. It's true. Soluble fiber can soak up enough water from your digestive tract to help firm up stool and slow its passage. While this remedy won't work for severe diarrhea, it may help mild or moderate cases.

Battles hemorrhoids. Fiber fights hemorrhoids by softening stools so they're easier to pass and relieving pressure on hemorrhoids.

Prevents gallstones. Soluble fiber soaks up cholesterol-containing bile salts, preventing their readsorption, while insoluble fiber helps food move through your small intestines to your colon more quickly, so bile has less time to sit in your gallbladder and form stones.

Lowers colon cancer risk. A soluble fiber called resistant starch passes undigested through your stomach and small intestine, but bacteria tackle it in your colon. That produces butyric acid, a fatty acid that helps prevent colon cancer. Good sources of resistant starch include black beans, kidney beans, peas, lentils, and unprocessed corn, sorghum, or barley. Soluble fiber also encourages a process in your large intestine that gets rid of certain bile acids that promote the growth of polyps that might become cancerous. On top of that, insoluble fiber speeds food through your digestive system, which might also help reduce your risk of colon cancer by eliminating cancer-causing substances quickly.

Diverts diverticulosis. People with low-fiber diets get diverticular disease more often than people who eat high-fiber foods. Low-fiber diets contribute to constipation and straining to have a bowel movement, which puts pressure on the intestinal lining. This can cause pouches, called diverticula, to form.

Chases away appendicitis. Burkitt suggested that appendicitis might be caused by chronic constipation and straining to pass small, hard stools that can lodge in your appendix and block its opening. He saw no cases of appendicitis in rural Africans who ate a high-fiber diet. Insoluble fiber speeds your food's passage through the digestive system to help prevent constipation.

Calms irritable bowel syndrome. Although insoluble fiber, like bran, may make IBS symptoms worse, the soluble fiber pectin may be very effective, helping improve symptoms, such as diarrhea.

How much fiber do you need after age 49? Experts recommend 30 grams of fiber a day for men and 21 grams for women. And you can go as high as 35 grams before fiber begins to interfere with your ability to absorb iron, calcium, zinc, and copper. However, most Americans get only 5 to 20 grams of fiber daily.

Halts hiatal hernia. A fiber-rich diet may keep you from developing a hiatal hernia, and associated heartburn, or making one worse. Straining from constipation is often blamed for causing hiatal hernia, but insoluble fiber keeps your stools soft and your bowels moving regularly.

Tames Crohn's disease. Soluble fiber, like pectin, may help relieve some symptoms of Crohn's, possibly by slowing and smoothing the passage of food through the intestines. Crohn's disease is much less prevalent in countries where most people eat a high-fiber diet.

Keeps ulcerative colitis at bay.
Psyllium, a type of soluble fiber, may help decrease ulcerative colitis flare-ups and relieve mild to moderate diarrhea.

Beyond digestion

Fiber doesn't just help digestive woes. It also helps safeguard you from other health problems.

High blood pressure. Some researchers think taking in 12 grams of soluble fiber every day might help lower high blood pressure.

Heart attacks and strokes. Soluble fiber in foods like carrots, lentils, oatmeal, and oat bran helps eliminate much of the artery-clogging cholesterol that can cause a heart attack or stroke. How? This type of fiber turns soft in your body, slowing things down in your stomach and small intestine. Soluble fiber sweeps cholesterol up and whisks it away, which helps lower the cholesterol levels in your blood. A study of 21,000 men in Finland found that those who ate an average of 35 grams of fiber a day had 25 percent fewer heart attacks than men who averaged just 16 grams a day.

Diabetes. Fiber helps your body absorb sugars and starches more slowly. This means your blood sugar rises gradually over a longer period, instead of skyrocketing after a meal. As a result, fiber keeps your blood sugar down.

Breast and prostate cancer. Although more research is needed, some studies suggest that eating a high-fiber diet might help reduce your risk of breast cancer or prostate cancer.

Weight gain. Like a sponge, fiber absorbs water and swells, making you feel full long after you eat it. As a result, you may eat less and skip fattening snacks and desserts. But that's not all. According to Burkitt,

Ask your doctor about psyl-lium supplements before taking them regularly, espe-cially if you take other medications. Psyllium could raise or lower your ability to absorb some drugs.

the more bulky, high-fiber foods you eat, the less fat you'll consume.

Varicose veins. Burkitt theorized that a low-fiber diet makes you more likely to strain during bowel move-ments. That could intensify the pressure on the veins in your legs, causing them to enlarge. He suggest-ed that eating high-fiber foods could help prevent varicose veins.

Impotency. Fiber-filled vegetables, like brussels spouts, navy beans, and zucchini, help maintain strong blood flow to the penis by lower-ing cholesterol and keeping your arteries clear.

8 things you should know about fiber

Fiber can help you in many ways. Here's how you can help fiber work wonders for you.

- ▸ *Start your day* with a whole-grain cereal, snack on raw veggies and fresh or dried fruits, substitute brown rice for white rice, and add beans to soups and stews.

- ▸ *Read cereal labels* to make sure you choose one with at least 5 grams of fiber per serving.

- ▸ *Check the ingredients list* of "whole grain" breads to make sure they're truly whole grain. You should see the word "whole" in the first ingredient. If the first ingredient is "enriched wheat flour," you aren't getting the full fiber and nutrient benefits of whole-grain bread.

- ▸ *Aim for a good mix* of soluble and insoluble fiber. Both types provide a variety of health benefits.

- ▸ *Avoid bran and citrus fruits* if you have IBS. Look for gentler sources of fiber, like peaches, apples, and cooked vegetables.

Rediscover super psyllium

Psyllium is the active ingredient in bulk laxatives, like Metamucil, Fiberall, Modane Bulk Powder, or Serutan. It helps keep your digestive tract healthy because it's a super source of water-soluble fiber. It's also herbal. "Psyllium" refers to tiny seeds from the perennial herb Plantago, or plantain. The oval seeds are odorless and nearly tasteless. Your body can't digest them, so they pass straight through, adding bulk to your stool. Psyllium seeds are coated in mucilage, which absorbs water in your intestines and lubricates your digestive tract.

The added bulk, extra water, and lubrication help stool move more effortlessly through your intestines. This also stimulates peristalsis, the muscular squeezing that pushes stool smoothly through your body. That means food passes through your colon more quickly, and bowel movements occur more easily and often. This is why psyllium can help relieve both temporary and chronic constipation.

Psyllium may also ease some symptoms of irritable bowel syndrome (IBS). Researchers in the Netherlands found only soluble forms of fiber, like psyllium, benefited IBS symptoms, including constipation. Insoluble fiber, the kind found in bran, did not. However, most people should also consume bran or other types of insoluble fiber with psyllium for optimal digestive health. Psyllium may also ease bowel movements for people with hemorrhoids and help prevent colon cancer, lower cholesterol, and heal anal fissures.

This gentle, natural laxative works overnight so you might decide to get out your orange juice and add some psyllium to it. Start with one dose a day, and gradually build up. Adding fiber too fast can cause gas and bloating. Don't take psyllium for more than a week without your doctor's approval. Take it with plenty of water, and don't take more than the recommended amount, or it may actually clog you up. See your doctor if you have bleeding or stomach pain two days after taking psyllium or if your constipation or diarrhea does not improve.

▶ ***Think food first.*** Foods are better for you and tastier than fiber supplements, which don't contain vital nutrients. Also, they can deplete your body of iron and calcium.

▶ ***Be creative.*** Add sliced bananas, peaches, or strawberries to yogurt, oatmeal, or cold cereal. Or dress up a sandwich with sliced carrots, green or red peppers, cucumbers, lettuce, or tomato.

▶ ***Discover the "wrapping."*** Whenever possible, wash fruits and veggies and eat the skin, as well as the tasty inside.

Water
Secret to tip-top digestion

Forget gold, diamonds, and oil. Plain old water is the most valuable substance on earth. Luckily, it's also the planet's most abundant liquid.

You could survive nearly a month without food, but only a few days without water. When it comes to your health, water makes a big splash. This essential liquid carries nutrients to every cell in your body, cushions your joints, and regulates your body temperature. Water is also important for digestion. It lubricates your digestive tract to keep it running smoothly. But that's just the beginning.

Healthy benefits

▶ Prevents constipation

▶ Relieves hemorrhoids

▶ Foils heartburn

▶ Lowers risk of colon cancer

▶ Wards off gallstones

▶ Combats dehydration

Conquers constipation. Water helps fiber soften stool and keep food moving through your digestive tract. This prevents constipation and hemorrhoids, and it may also help anal fissures heal. When you increase your fiber intake, especially if taking a psyllium supplement, be sure to drink plenty of water to prevent an intestinal blockage.

Fights heartburn. Water washes acid out of your esophagus and dilutes it in your stomach to prevent heartburn. For best results, drink a glass of water either an hour before or after meals, rather than with them. This could also protect you from Barrett's esophagus, which sometimes leads to esophageal cancer.

Outsmarts colon cancer. This natural cancer fighter washes away or dilutes cancer-causing substances to help protect you from colon cancer. A small study in Taiwan found that men who drank the most water lowered their risk of developing colon cancer by 92 percent, compared with men who drank very little water.

Deters gallstones. Drinking water helps ward off gallstones. It helps the bile in your liver dissolve cholesterol that could become painful gallstones.

If your digestive system is plagued with problems, make water a priority. Whether it's constipation, heartburn, gas, irritable bowel syndrome, or just plain indigestion, water will soothe your system and get things moving in the right direction.

Beyond digestion

Water can also heal your body, moisturize your skin, and help you control your weight. But this amazing substance doesn't stop there.

Dehydration. Drinking an appropriate amount of water every day (enough to produce a quart of urine per day is about right) helps prevent

Word to the wise

Thirst isn't always the best indicator of dehydration. As you get older, your body loses its ability to make you thirsty. Some medications also dull your sense of thirst. Dehydration causes almost 7 percent of hospitalizations among older adults. Watch out for these warning signs:

▸ dry lips and mouth

▸ dizziness or headaches

▸ forgetfulness or confusion

▸ rapid breathing

▸ increased heart rate

▸ dark urine or constipation

▸ weakness or lack of energy

dehydration. Just remember — if you have diarrhea or vomiting, you may also need to replenish your electrolytes. Electrolytes are salts and minerals normally found in blood, tissue fluids, and cells. Loss of electrolytes can cause serious problems. Most people get enough electrolytes from salt in their food and other dietary sources. Morton Lite Salt Mixture contains only half as much sodium chloride per serving as regular salt. The other half is potassium chloride, giving a better balance of these two important electrolytes for most people than regular salt. You can also get electrolytes by trying this inexpensive method used in underdeveloped countries — drink the cooled water left in the pot after cooking rice.

If you're sick, or especially after you have surgery, drinking water is an easy way to put yourself back on the road to recovery. After surgery, your body retains water to help it heal, so adding to your supply gives your body an extra boost just when it needs it most.

Heart and artery disease. When you drink water, it becomes absorbed in your blood. This makes your blood less thick and less likely to clot.

Kidney stones. A five-year Italian study of people who had kidney stones found that the ones who drank lots of water only developed half as many kidney stones. If you're at risk of kidney stones, make water your first line of defense.

About three-quarters of your body is made up of water, including 83 percent of your blood. Even if you're a couch potato, you lose up to 10 cups a day, through sweat, urine, and even breathing. If you're active, you lose even more.

Arthritis. If you have arthritis, or gout — a form of arthritis — drink plenty of water. Water cushions and lubricates your joints, making them less painful. This refreshing drink also helps dilute and flush out uric acid, which causes gout.

UTIs. Water is one of your best bets to prevent urinary tract infections. It helps flush out your urinary tract, taking bacteria with it.

The danger of drinking too much water

A recent study of Boston marathon runners found that endurance athletes can drink so much water they dilute their electrolytes, a condition called water intoxication. The researchers estimated that more than 10 percent of the runners had mild cases. Severe cases are rarer but may be life threatening. The researchers also found that weight gain during the marathon was a key sign of the problem.

During exercise, sports and health organizations recommend drinking when you are thirsty. Don't guzzle large amounts of water or sports drinks before exercising to get a jump on the water you'll lose by sweating.

In at least one case, a 45-year-old woman developed water intoxication by drinking large quantities of water to suppress her appetite. Even during heavy exertion in high heat, the U.S. Army has warned its members against drinking more than six 8-ounce glasses of water per hour or more than 48 8-ounce glasses in 12 hours.

Obesity. Water has no fat, sugar, or calories, making it the perfect drink for dieters. Try a refreshing glass before eating. Water fills you up, so you'll eat less.

Dry skin. Water is critical for healthy skin. Both water in the air and the water you drink gives shape and nourishment to your cells. It makes your skin elastic and supple, instead of dried up like a prune. And don't forget what it does for your lips. Water keeps them moist and kissably soft.

7 things you should know about water

How much water do you really need? When should you use bottled water instead of tap water? These handy guidelines provide all the answers.

▸ *Aim for the equivalent of eight 8-ounce glasses* of water a day. New research suggests you can get some of that from water-containing foods, like soup, tea, juice, milk, fruits, and vegetables. Drink extra water on the days you exercise. But the bottom line is how much urine you void each day. Less than a quart of urine per day means you probably need to drink more water.

▸ *Beware of drinking* tap water when traveling to underdeveloped countries. The water supply is often contaminated with bacteria. Use bottled water for drinking and brushing your teeth. Don't use ice unless you know it was made from boiled or filtered water.

▸ *Choose either tap or bottled water.* Tap water is generally purified with chlorine, which can leave a flavor or odor behind. Bottled water is often filtered, or treated with ultraviolet light or a form of oxygen. These methods sometimes make bottled water taste "cleaner" than chlorinated tap water.

▸ *Take precautions* if you reuse water bottles. Wash them with hot, soapy water to keep bacteria from building up.

▸ *Drink more water during hot weather.* You might also need more water if you're over age 70, drink alcohol, or have increased your intake of fiber, protein, salt, or sugar.

▸ *Know your body's needs.* Diabetes, kidney disease, burns, blood loss, diarrhea, vomiting, fever, or taking diuretics increases your body's need for water.

▸ *Consider your environment.* Spending time at high altitudes, whether on the ground or in a plane, usually means you need more water.

Exercise
Walk to calm digestive woes

You're in for an eye-opening surprise if you think exercise can't do much for your digestive system. Take a look at these benefits.

Beats constipation. A brisk walk every day, or any other moderate exercise, can ease constipation without the side effects of harsh laxatives. Preventing constipation may also lower your risk of diverticular disease, hemorrhoids, hiatal hernias, and even varicose veins.

Deflates gas and bloating. Moving your body speeds up digestion and helps gas pass quickly through your digestive system. It can also strengthen your abdominal muscles to ease bloating.

Extinguishes heartburn. Anxiety and stress can bring on heartburn, but regular exercise is a champion stress fighter. Battle stress and heartburn at the same time by being more active.

> ## Healthy benefits
> ▶ Eases constipation
> ▶ Calms heartburn
> ▶ Gets rid of gas
> ▶ Fights bloating
> ▶ Quiets ulcers
> ▶ Helps manage IBS
> ▶ Heads off hemorrhoids
> ▶ Cuts odds of colon cancer
> ▶ Trims gallstone risk
> ▶ Tames inflammatory bowel disease

Soothes ulcers. Stress doesn't cause ulcers, but it may trigger pain if you have one. Try walking or other exercise to see if that lessens your stress and makes you feel better.

Relieves irritable bowel syndrome. Physical activity may help ease symptoms of irritable bowel syndrome.

Fends off colon cancer. According to one study, regular physical activity may slash your risk of colon cancer by an amazing 83 percent. Too much weight can boost your colon cancer risk, but exercise can help you shed pounds and lower your risk.

Chases away gallstones. Getting enough exercise may trim your risk of gallstones.

Tames Crohn's and ulcerative colitis. Physical activity helps your intestines work better. It also relaxes you and works off the stress and tension that affect your digestive system. While stress may not cause digestive diseases like Crohn's and ulcerative colitis, studies show it can trigger attacks and make symptoms worse.

You can look forward to health benefits even if you only rack up 30 minutes of moderate activity each day. In fact, if you're just starting to become more active, take your exercise in 10-minute portions. Start with three sessions a day. Soon you'll be able to do 30 minutes of moderate activity all at once. You'll know it's moderate if it causes you to breathe hard but lets you talk without gasping for breath.

For winning results, experts suggest you aim for 30 minutes of exercise at least three days a week. If you can move up to four days or more, you might get even better results, and your digestive system will thank you.

Before you begin any exercise program, talk with your doctor about the best activities for you. Ask these questions.

▶ Is it safe for me to do the exercises I have planned?

▶ How can I find out whether I'm exercising hard enough?

▶ How can I avoid exercising too hard?

▶ Are there any sports or exercises I should avoid?

▶ Do I have any health conditions or take any medications that could affect my exercise plans?

Beyond digestion

Exercise adds more to your life than good digestion. It keeps your body functioning like a well-oiled machine and helps you fend off a variety of ills like these.

Heart disease. Walking may be the best and least expensive way to a healthy heart. It lowers your blood pressure, cuts cholesterol, and strengthens your circulatory system. In fact, you may slash your heart attack risk in half just by walking 30 to 45 minutes three times a week.

Stroke. Moderate activity perks up your circulation, which can prevent blood clots that lead to brain attacks, or strokes.

Breast cancer. Exercising regularly may help you dodge breast cancer, and it's never too late to start. One study found that women who began exercising after menopause dropped their breast cancer risk by 40 percent. Most surprising of all, activities like gardening and household chores protected them more than aerobics and weight lifting.

Osteoporosis. Doing 45 minutes of weight lifting activities twice a week strengthens your muscles and bones and improves balance, which can help limit falls, stave off osteoporosis, and protect your bones from fractures. Moderate exercise can even improve symptoms of knee osteoarthritis.

Colds and flu. Brisk walking, or other moderate exercise, keeps your immune system in tip-top condition by stimulating natural killer cells that attack viruses and bacteria.

Depression. Exercise may relieve depression as well as some medications, according to a Duke University study. Something as simple as gardening could dig you out of the dumps. However, don't stop taking antidepressants or any medication without consulting your doctor.

Exercise can also:

- fight fatigue
- help you lose weight
- preserve memory and mental alertness
- defeat insomnia
- protect against prostate cancer

9 things you should know about exercise

Forget about the gung-ho fitness experts on TV. You don't have to be like them to get more active. Instead, take advantage of these hints to choose fitness that fits you.

- *Focus on activities* like walking, yard work, playing with kids, and housework. They are all convenient forms of exercise that are also free.

▶ **Start slow** so achy muscles or injuries don't leave you discouraged. You can always add more vigorous and interesting exercises later.

▶ **Warm up** for 10 minutes before you exercise to protect your heart and other muscles. To warm up, gradually begin whatever activity you'll be doing. At the end of your workout, cool down by slowing your pace for about five to 10 minutes. This will bring your heart rate and breathing back to normal. Finish with some stretches to prevent stiffness.

▶ **Sneak extra activity** into your day. When you're shopping, park farther from the store, or walk around while talking on a cordless phone.

▶ **Try to wait** at least two hours after a meal before you exercise. You'll enjoy your workout more when you don't feel full, and you'll avoid cramps and other problems.

▶ **Learn from a class** or instructor to make sure you know how to do new exercises correctly. With a little research, you can probably find a class for free.

▶ **Take up fun forms** of exercise, like dancing, tennis, or golf.

▶ **Beat bad weather** by walking in the mall or renting a home fitness video.

▶ **Drink water** as you exercise to replace the fluids you lose through sweat.

Probiotics
Friendly bacteria to the rescue

Your digestive system is home to billions of bacteria. Most of them are harmless, and many actually keep you healthy. These good guys are known as probiotics, and you need them to digest food, fight off illness, and maintain a healthy gut.

These beneficial organisms have antibiotic and anti-inflammatory powers. They kill infectious bacteria and protect the delicate lining along your digestive tract from attack by disease-causing organisms. They even boost your immune system by helping your body make antibodies and phagocytes, germ-killing cells.

Unfortunately, the good bacteria sometimes die off, throwing your digestive system out of balance. A round of antibiotics, a poor diet, or illness may kill many of the helpful "bugs," creating the perfect opportunity for harmful ones to invade and take over.

An overgrowth of bad bacteria can quickly lead to diarrhea, ulcers, or more serious chronic conditions, such as inflammatory bowel disease (IBD).

Healthy benefits
▶ Treats diarrhea
▶ Fends off ulcers
▶ Eases lactose intolerance
▶ Helps relieve ulcerative colitis and Crohn's disease
▶ Soothes diverticulitis
▶ Defends against gastritis
▶ Helps prevent colon cancer
▶ Prevents pouchitis

Regain control of your gut by adding back the good guys. Probiotic supplements and foods with added probiotics, like Dannon's cultured dairy drink, DanActive, contain live bacteria similar to the good ones that inhabit your gut. Adding them to your diet every day floods your intestines with beneficial bacteria that remain active in your digestive tract.

The benefits can be very real. For instance, if you suffer inflammation of the stomach, or an intestinal or urinary tract infection, maybe you should drink *acidophilus* milk right away — and every day. Often added to yogurt and milk, this friendly bacterium defends against gastritis, or inflammation of the stomach, intestinal infections from parasites, and even urinary tract infections, and it may ease the symptoms of diverticulitis and IBD by reducing intestinal inflammation.

Talk with your doctor to find out if probiotics could relieve your digestive problems. The biggest and perhaps only downside to probiotic therapy — you may have to take them indefinitely for long-term benefits. The payoff, however, may be well worth it.

Treats diarrhea. Studies show *acidophilus* effectively treats traveler's diarrhea caused by *E. coli* infections, as well as diarrhea triggered by antibiotics and radiation therapy.

Short-circuits colon cancer. *Acidophilus* holds promise in preventing colon cancer, too. Experts suspect, among other things, it boosts your immune system, suppresses the growth of cancer-causing cells, and binds cancer-causing agents in your intestines before they create trouble.

Eases lactose intolerance. *Acidophilus* also predigests the sugar lactose, so dairy foods made with *acidophilus* may be easier to tolerate if you are lactose intolerant. Two other bacteria, *Lactobacillus bulgaricus* and *Streptococcus thermophilus* may do an even better job of predigesting lactose.

Thwarts ulcers. The beneficial bacterium *bifidus* found in yogurt and buttermilk is also naturally present in your digestive tract. Together with *acidophilus* it may help control the growth of *H. pylori*, the organism that often causes stomach ulcers.

Word to the wise

You may experience temporary gas and bloating when you first increase your intake of probiotics. However, if you take probiotics on a regular basis, these symptoms should fade as your body adjusts.

Curbs inflammatory bowel disease. You probably never thought *E. coli* could be good for you, but one strain is — Nissle 1917 found in the probiotic product Mutaflor. It's one of the beneficial bacteria scientists say may help maintain remission in IBD.

Battles ulcerative colitis. The probiotic supplement VSL#3 contains several kinds of bacteria for a power-packed punch — four strains of *Lactobacillus*, three strains of *Bifidobacterium*, and one of *Streptococci*. Studies so far show it works. In one recent clinical trial, 20 people with ulcerative colitis in remission took 3 grams of VSL#3 twice a day. After one year, 15 of them remained in remission.

The digestive tract in a healthy adult is home to 5 to 8 pounds of bacteria numbering in the trillions — most of them beneficial.

Outwits Crohn's disease. Another study found VSL#3 helped Crohn's disease sufferers. People with Crohn's who took the supplement for a year had only a 20-percent risk of relapse compared to those on the prescription drug mesalamine, the standard treatment for IBD.

Nips pouchitis in the bud. VSL#3 may also prevent pouchitis, a complication occurring in half the people who undergo surgery to remove their large intestine.

8 things you should know about probiotics

Boosting your intake of live bacteria is easy. Just try this advice for picking and storing probiotic products.

- ▸ *Look for labels* saying "contains live cultures," "contains bacteria," or "promotes healthy digestion." Some products might not use the word "probiotic."

- ▸ *Read labels* to find out exactly which bacteria a food or supplement contains.

- ▸ *Shop for the supplement VSL#3* at high-quality health food stores and pharmacies, or buy it on the Internet at *www.vsl3.com*.

- ▸ *Aim to get* at least 1 billion probiotic bacteria a day. Products may list 1 billion as 10^9 or 1×10^9.

- ▸ *Check the expiration date.* Only living bacteria benefit your gut, and the older the product gets, the fewer bacteria are alive.

- ▸ *Pick products* that list the expected amount of bacteria alive at time of use, rather than at the time of manufacture. In a recent lab test, those listing time of use tended to contain more living bacteria.

Another way to keep your gut healthy

Probiotics are the good bacteria that live in your intestines. Prebiotics are the nutrients they eat, carbohydrates your body can't digest, sometimes called resistant "starch."

One type of prebiotic is a carbohydrate called fructooligosaccharide (FOS). Your body doesn't have the enzymes needed to digest FOS as it moves through your digestive tract, but the beneficial bacteria in your colon do.

Once the FOS reaches them, they break it down and feed on it. Prebiotics, such as FOS, make a perfect meal for hungry, helpful bacteria, like *bifidobacteria* and *lactobacilli*. Scientists say adding just a small amount of prebiotics to your daily diet can stimulate the growth of these friendly bacteria in your intestines, plus provide benefits of their own. Inulin, a kind of FOS, may help relieve both constipation and diarrhea.

Surprisingly, prebiotics are easy to find in everyday foods. Inulin and oligofructose, two of the most well-studied ones, are found naturally in many fruits, vegetables, and whole grains. You can even get prebiotics from processed foods, such as yogurt, ice cream, chocolate, candy, butter, and breakfast cereals. Expect to see inulin listed as an ingredient on food labels in the near future. These are just a few of the foods packed with prebiotics.

- wheat bran and oats, barley, rye, flaxseed, and other whole grains
- chicory, sometimes added to coffee or used as a coffee substitute
- asparagus and artichokes, as well as leeks, garlic, and onions
- greens, including collard and mustard greens, as well as spinach,
- fruit, such as berries and bananas
- legumes, including lentils, kidney beans, navy beans, chickpeas

If you have a weakened immune system, talk with your doctor before loading up on pre- or probiotics.

▸ **Store probiotic foods or supplements** in the refrigerator to keep bacteria alive and extend their shelf life.

▸ **Wait at least two hours** after taking an antibiotic before you take a probiotic.

Sleep
'Hit the sack' to soothe digestion

"I can't believe I ate the whole thing," moans bathrobe-clad Ralph in the famous old Alka-Seltzer commercial. Most of us have experienced a night when digestive troubles kept sleep away, but you might be surprised to learn that the opposite is true. A good night's sleep may help prevent digestive distress.

Repels ulcers. According to researchers, you may raise your odds of developing ulcers just by being awake long after midnight. What's more, the problem could start during the day. What you eat and drink can cause tiny amounts of damage to your stomach. That damage may add up over time and grow into an ulcer.

Healthy benefits
▸ Helps prevent ulcers
▸ Calms irritable bowel syndrome

So why don't we all have ulcers? Fortunately, the body seems to have a built-in damage control system. Experts believe special proteins, called TFF2, help repair your stomach lining. Although these proteins exist naturally in your stomach most of the time, their amounts can rise up to 300 percent during normal sleep. So you might just snooze your way to a healthier stomach — especially from 1 a.m. to 5 a.m.

Tames irritable bowel syndrome. Lack of shut-eye has also been linked to irritable bowel syndrome (IBS) in women. A two-month study found that IBS symptoms could be worse after nights when you don't get enough sleep. Just one night is all it takes.

A larger study focused on IBS, frequent heartburn, and frequent indigestion in people who reported sleep disturbances. The scientists found that over 30 percent of the participants had IBS, while at least 20 percent had frequent indigestion. They also learned that IBS was more common in people reporting sleep disturbances than in those who didn't.

And yet, scientists still aren't sure whether IBS leads to sleep disturbances or sleep disturbances contribute to IBS, or perhaps they're both caused by the same thing. However, the body uses sleep to make many types of repairs, and it's possible that a good night's sleep might help repair digestive problems. More research is needed to find out, but meanwhile getting extra sleep could still do your digestive system good.

Missing sleep may also weaken your immune system. That's the last thing you want if there's a stomach virus going around, or if you need help from your immune system to dodge digestive problems.

Word to the wise

Your spouse complains that you snort, gasp, or make choking sounds during sleep, but you don't remember any of that. Don't ignore these key signs of sleep apnea, a potentially life-threatening disease that deprives you of oxygen during sleep and may lead to a heart attack or stroke. People with sleep apnea have higher-than-average rates of car accidents, possibly because they suffer from daytime sleepiness. See your doctor for treatment.

Losing more than the occasional few nights of sleep is becoming common. According to the National Sleep Foundation's 2005 Sleep in America poll, about half of the people interviewed said they get a good night's sleep almost every night. Another quarter of the interviewees sleep well just a few nights a week, while the rest only meet their sleep needs a few nights a month, or less.

For most people, getting more sleep is just a matter of planning, but others can't get a good night's sleep no matter how hard they try. This sleep disturbance could be insomnia. Symptoms include trouble falling asleep, waking frequently during the night, waking up too early without being able to go back to sleep, and waking up feeling unrested.

Quiet insomnia with melatonin

People with sleep problems, particularly older adults, may find help from melatonin. Melatonin is a hormone produced by the pineal gland located at the base of your brain. It regulates your body clock's natural wake-sleep cycle. Some evidence suggests melatonin levels tend to drop as you get older. By increasing your body's natural supply, you may get a better night's sleep — the truly restful kind of sleep associated with restoration and repair.

In one study, 372 people with insomnia over age 55 were checked for how much melatonin they excreted. The researchers found that 30 percent expelled below-normal levels of the hormone. Although all study participants took 2 milligrams of melatonin every night for three weeks, these 112 people benefited more than the others.

You can increase your melatonin naturally by eating whole grains, legumes, nuts, milk, meat, fish, poultry, or eggs about an hour before bedtime. These foods contain the amino acid tryptophan, which the body can convert to melatonin. You can also eat foods that contain melatonin, like oats, sweet corn, rice, ginger, cherries, tomatoes, bananas, and barley.

Check with your doctor before trying melatonin supplements. They're not right for everyone and can have unpleasant side effects, such as grogginess during the day. Nevertheless, melatonin may be better for you than sleep-promoting drugs. If your doctor gives you the green light, you may want to experiment to find out what works. The fast-release melatonin supplements will get into your bloodstream quicker, and the slow-release pills will keep the hormone at a more even level throughout the night.

Many people have insomnia occasionally. But if you have persistent insomnia, see your doctor to make sure it's not a sign of sleep apnea, especially if you also experience morning headaches, snoring, or tingling of the legs.

11 things you should know about sleep

Imagine a relaxing scene to resist sleep-robbing stress, and you may find yourself falling asleep. Researchers found a waterfall scene effective, but you might prefer the rhythmic sounds of waves on a beach or the beauty of the mountains. For even better results, try these sleep-promoting ideas.

▶ *Get a little sunshine in the morning.* Morning sunshine increases the level of melatonin in your body at night when you need it. This hormone helps regulate your sleep cycle naturally.

▶ *Keep a sleep diary for several weeks.* Note when and how long you sleep, when you sleep well, when you don't, and when you feel sleepy. Also, track your health habits. Either use a notebook or visit *www.sleepfoundation.org* and use their interactive Web diary.

▶ *Cut back on caffeine or eliminate it.* Check medicine labels for caffeine, too.

▶ *Get regular exercise.* About 20 to 30 minutes of exercise three or four days a week could improve your snooze time

Circadian rhythms, your body's internal clock, controls when you sleep and wake. That clock can get "out of sync" with real time as you age. As a result, older adults may get sleepy long before bedtime and wake well before sunrise.

▶ *Ask your doctor* whether any medicine you take could cause insomnia.

▶ *Keep your bedroom dark,* quiet, and cool.

▶ *Relax during the half hour before bed.* Try a warm bath.

▶ *Go to bed at the same time every night* and get up at your regular time every morning, even on weekends.

- *Use your bedroom for sleep,* not watching television, eating, or working.

- *Avoid alcohol,* exercise, heavy meals, nicotine, and large amounts of liquids during the evening.

- *Don't try to sleep with cold hands or feet.* Wear socks or gloves to warm them.

Stress management
How to calm a gut reaction

You're enjoying a leisurely hike through a scenic forest when, suddenly, a massive bear blocks your path — and he looks very hungry. Your body immediately triggers its "emergency response system."

- First, you freeze so you won't stumble into the bear's clutches.

- Next, you throw your lunch at the bear and sprint away.

- Finally, when you're safe, you catch your breath, calm down, and try to recover.

Healthy benefits

- Foils stress-induced diarrhea
- Ambushes heartburn
- Cuts ulcer risk
- Inhibits bloating
- Eases IBS symptoms
- Reduces IBS flare-ups

You may have lost your lunch but, thanks to your emergency response system, you didn't become lunch. Your emergency response system is called the general adaptation syndrome. It has three stages, and it affects your whole body, including your digestive system.

When you spotted the bear, the fight-or-flight stage kicked in. Adrenaline started pumping, and your body switched to crisis mode so you could react quickly. After you stopped moving, stage two started, and your body generated resources to help you resolve the crisis. The final rest and recovery stage happened after you escaped and knew you were safe.

Your digestive system responded immediately when fight-or-flight was triggered.

▸ Your mouth went dry.

▸ Your stomach produced more acid.

▸ The muscle action that moves waste through your gut sped up.

▸ Secretions of digestive enzymes were cut back or stopped.

You should ease back to normal once you reach the third stage, but that doesn't always happen. Your body reacts to job and home stresses the same way it does to life-or-death situations. What's more, if frequent stress keeps your body on alert too much, wear-and-tear sets in. Learn to manage your stress, and you might find digestive relief.

Banishes bloating. If you're under stress, you're more likely to swallow extra air, which causes bloating. Seek out relaxing ways to lower your stress levels, and you might stop bloating before it starts.

Silences inflammatory bowel disease. If you have Crohn's disease or ulcerative colitis, stress management might help you stay in remission. Studies suggest that stress may make symptom flare-ups more likely.

Defeats diarrhea. Stress can directly trigger a bout of diarrhea. Later in this chapter, you'll learn ways to control your reaction to stress to help you prevent your next episode.

Battles ulcers. Stress may not cause ulcers, but it might increase your risk of developing them. If you already have an ulcer, stress could make it worse. Learn what best helps you to deal with stress. This keeps your stomach from making too much stomach acid, and that gives ulcers a chance to heal.

Subdues irritable bowel syndrome. People with irritable bowel syndrome (IBS) may have a colon problem that makes their intestines more sensitive to stress. That's why IBS can make your insides feel tied up in knots. Fortunately, relaxing, natural remedies can quickly smooth out the kinks and soothe intestinal problems.

A research review by the Agency for Healthcare Research and Quality found some evidence that relaxation therapies may help relieve digestive tract disorders. But that's not all.

According to the American College of Gastroenterology (ACG) Functional Gastrointestinal Disorders Task Force, behavioral therapies, like relaxation techniques, may benefit people with IBS. Although more and better research is needed, the task force still recommends relaxation as a treatment worth considering. Meanwhile, the ACG already advocates including stress management as part of treatment for functional abdominal pain syndrome.

Scientists even offer a reason why easing your mind could soothe your gut. They call it the brain-gut axis. Your digestive tract has almost as many nerve cells in it as your spinal cord. In fact, your digestive tract constantly trades information with your central nervous system. So if you're stressed, don't be surprised if your digestive system shows the strain. And if you relax, your digestive tract may feel better, too.

Word to the wise

A high-stress day calls for extra stress management, but some popular stress reducers could sabotage your efforts. So should you spend your last dregs of energy on your usual exercise workout or just unwind with a glass of wine and a relaxing evening of mindless TV? Stick with the workout. A study from the University of Illinois Urbana-Champaign suggests that idle relaxing isn't as stress-reducing as a good workout. What's more, drinking alcohol can interfere with the deep, restful sleep you need to face tomorrow's stressors. Next time, remember to ditch the alcohol and swing into an anxiety-whipping workout.

12 things you should know about stress management

Control stress and you'll help protect yourself from heart and prostate disease, build up your immune system, ditch insomnia, relieve inflammatory bowel disease and maybe more. Try these easy and relaxing solutions to manage your stress.

▸ *Walk off stress* and put digestive pain on the run. Walking is aerobic exercise — the kind that produces brain chemicals to perk up your mood and mental well-being.

▸ *Learn from Lou Gehrig and Jimmy Stewart* and deal with stress or sadness. Lower blood pressure, fewer ulcers, and less colitis are just some of the potential benefits of letting yourself cry when you need to.

▸ *Reduce stress with laughter*. Hunt for the humor in stressful situations. Read funny books and watch amusing movies or TV shows.

▸ *Write in a journal* or diary.

▸ *Revamp that to-do list* and shake off stress. Overstuffing your schedule multiplies anxiety. Make a list of your daily tasks. Rate how important each activity is. Cut out the lowest rated tasks.

▸ *Listen* to relaxing music.

▸ *Say a prayer.* Praying might improve your ability to deal with stress, and you may find other benefits in prayer, too.

▸ *Try this breathing exercise.* Put one hand on your stomach. Inhale slowly and deeply while counting from one to four. Exhale as you count backward from four to one.

▸ *Stop skimping* on sleep.

▸ *Grab a cereal bowl.* British research suggests that breakfast eaters feel less stressed than people who skip breakfast.

▸ *Try gardening.*

▸ *Take all your vacation days* this year and see how your stress and your stomach improve.

Unsaturated fats
Trim health risks with good fats

Just like Rodney Dangerfield, fat gets no respect. Dieters and others concerned with their health avoid it like the plague.

Sometimes that's not a bad idea. Too much saturated fat, found in animal products like meat, whole milk, cheese, and butter, increases your risk for heart disease, stroke, diabetes, and cancer. But you shouldn't lump all fats in with this nutrition villain.

Healthy benefits

▶ Prevents heartburn

▶ Cuts colon cancer risk

▶ Wipes out ulcer-causing bacteria

▶ Helps prevent gastritis

▶ Lowers risk of gallstones

▶ Fights relapses of Crohn's disease

▶ Reduces stomach cancer risk

In fact, some types of fat are essential for good health. Polyunsaturated fats, along with monounsaturated fats, the kind found in olive oil, canola oil, peanuts, and avocados, belong in this category.

Omega-3 and omega-6 fatty acids are the two main types of polyunsaturated fat. Fish, fish oil, walnuts, flaxseed, and canola provide omega-3, while you can find omega-6 in vegetable oils like corn, safflower, soybean, cottonseed, and sunflower. However, the typical diet contains 20 times as much omega-6, which promotes inflammation, as omega-3. Therefore, it's good to decrease omega-6 consumption and increase omega-3 consumption.

Even Jack Sprat would change his stance on fat if he knew all the ways these unsaturated fats help your body. For instance, monounsaturated fats lower bad LDL cholesterol while boosting your levels of good HDL cholesterol. They also fill you up so you eat less. Since being overweight contributes to heartburn, you can drop pounds and ditch heartburn with these good fats. Omega-3 lowers LDL and triglyceride levels and fights inflammation, arthritis, and even depression. Like omega-3 and monounsaturated fats, omega-6 fatty acids lower LDL, but unfortunately, they also bring down beneficial HDL levels.

When it comes to digestive problems, unsaturated fats certainly pull their weight. Here's how:

Guards against ulcers and gastritis. Polyunsaturated fats may wipe out *H. pylori,* the bacteria that cause stomach ulcers, gastritis, and sometimes even stomach cancer.

Outsmarts gallstones. A high intake of unsaturated fats reduces your risk of developing gallstones.

Curbs colon cancer. Fish oil, rich in omega-3, may protect against colon cancer. Studies with rats show fish oil affects the fatty acid composition of cell membranes, which affects whether a cell becomes cancerous. Studies also show that olive oil, one of the best sources of monounsaturated fat, may reduce the risk of some cancers, including colon and rectal cancer. It may protect against breast, prostate, and esophageal cancers, too.

Calms Crohn's disease. Fish oil may also help people with Crohn's disease. A study of Crohn's disease sufferers shows the anti-inflammatory properties of fish oil can reduce the number of relapses. Check with your doctor about fish oil supplements, or add fish oil to your diet naturally by eating salmon, tuna, mackerel, sardines, anchovies, and herring.

The polyunsaturated fats omega-3 and omega-6 are called essential fatty acids. Your body needs them but can't produce them on its own, so you must get them through your diet.

Helps halt heartburn. Being overweight may cause the valve that prevents heartburn to malfunction. A Harvard study found that avoiding saturated fats and keeping total

Benefits of fish outweigh risks

Be smart about eating seafood, but don't cut back on eating this delicious food that's full of healthy omega-3 fatty acids. Although some types of fish have become the main food sources of contaminants, like mercury and polychlorinated biphenyls (PCBs), most people don't eat enough fish to be in danger of mercury poisoning. According to the Department of Health and Human Services and the Environmental Protection Agency (EPA), you should avoid these four types of fish — shark, swordfish, king mackerel, and tilefish — because they are high in mercury. Limit your intake of albacore tuna and tuna steak to one serving a week. Enjoy fish that are low in mercury, like shrimp, salmon, catfish, and light canned tuna. Pregnant women can eat up to 12 ounces (two meals) a week of a variety of low-mercury fish and shellfish. You can learn ways to avoid PCBs and other toxins in *Salmon* in Chapter 5.

fat intake under 30 percent might help people lose weight better than a strict low-fat diet. The Harvard diet also recommends getting more of the healthier unsaturated fats, such as the omega-3 fatty acids in fish, flaxseed, and walnuts, and the monounsaturated fats in nuts, peanut butter, and olives.

Remember, no matter how healthy a fat may be, all fats pack a whopping nine calories per gram, as opposed to four calories per gram of protein or carbohydrate. Experts say to limit all fat to 30 percent of your total calories. No more than 10 percent should come from saturated fat.

Another thing to keep in mind is the ratio of your omega-6 to omega-3 fatty acids. Too much omega-6 and not enough omega-3 can lead to all sorts of health problems, like headaches, arthritis, asthma, and arrhythmia.

Word to the wise

Not all unsaturated fats are good for your colon. Studies show that olive oil, rich in monounsaturated fat, and fish oil, loaded with omega-3 fatty acids, may protect against colon cancer. On the other hand, corn oil, a source of omega-6 linoleic acid, seems to promote it.

2 things you should know about unsaturated fats

Look for ways to replace saturated fats with healthier unsaturated fats. Also, remember to aim for a better ratio of omega-6 to omega-3 fatty acids.

▸ *Eliminate deep-fried foods,* margarine, and salad dressings made with corn oil or soybean oil. Replace corn or soybean oil with canola or olive oil.

▸ *Substitute avocado* for cheese in a veggie sandwich.

CHAPTER 5

"GARBAGE IN, GARBAGE OUT," CLAIMED THE OLD COMPUTER PROVERB. It meant that poor quality

Diet additions to aid digestion

input led to a poor final result. The same is true with your body. Put bad food in and you'll get bad health out. But once you know the best foods to feed your digestive system, your body may thank you with remarkable improvements in digestive ills and overall digestive health.

Apples
Super fruit keeps you healthy

Everyone likes a package deal. That description fits an apple. Wrapped in a thin, tough, colorful skin is one of the most delicious, nutritious foods to be found anywhere.

One medium apple has it all — 5 grams of fiber, 170 milligrams of potassium, no fat or sodium — and all for only 80 calories. What's more, it stores well and is always in season.

Apples are packed with antioxidants — cancer-fighting free-radical scavengers like vitamin C, phenolic acids, and flavonoids. These valuable phytonutrients are found in the skin, the flesh, and the core. Quercetin, one of the apple's flavonoids, has even more anti-cancer power than the potent antioxidant vitamin C. Snack on an apple every day to reap these benefits.

Healthy benefits

▶ Prevents and helps cure constipation

▶ Relieves diarrhea

▶ Fends off hemorrhoids

▶ Guards against diverticulosis

▶ Wards off hiatal hernia

▶ Inhibits appendicitis

▶ Helps lower colon cancer risk

Curbs constipation. Are your bowels too sluggish — or too speedy? Either way, this super fruit is sure to help. Apples are loaded with dietary fiber. It helps curb your appetite, promotes a longer-lasting sense of fullness after meals, and slows the digestion and absorption of carbohydrates. Eighty percent of the apple's fiber is the kind called pectin. This remarkable soluble fiber absorbs water and provides bulk and moisture in your digestive tract. It also provides welcome relief for digestive problems ranging from constipation to diarrhea.

Resists diarrhea. Applesauce is a great diarrhea remedy. Since the insoluble fiber peel has been removed, the soluble pectin in applesauce gently helps congeal and solidify loose stools. But once diarrhea is gone, eat that peel. Lots of phytonutrient punch, and the constipation-relieving effect of insoluble fiber, is lost when an apple is peeled. About half of the vitamin C is found just beneath the skin.

Prevents "pressure diseases." An apple peel provides insoluble fiber — a natural way to prevent chronic constipation. The late Dr. Denis Burkitt, author of *Eat Right — To Stay Healthy and Enjoy Life More*, identified fiber-depleted diets and associated constipation as the common cause behind "pressure diseases" like appendicitis, diverticular disease, hemorrhoids, and hiatal hernias. But these aren't likely to be a big threat to regular eaters of unpeeled apples.

Snubs colon cancer. The fiber in apples may also help eliminate cancer-causing substances from your bowels. "When diets are rich in dietary fiber," Burkitt said, "the stools passed are usually large. If carcinogens (substances that produce cancer) are diluted in a large volume of stool and also if they are discarded out of the bowel fairly quickly (as happens with fiber-rich diets) rather than hanging around, they will be less dangerous."

Word to the wise

Beware of unpasteurized apple juice and cider. They can look, taste, and smell delicious but still transport dangerous E. coli, bacteria that cause dangerous food poisoning.

Burkitt's cultural studies also showed that more animal fat in diets was associated with a higher incidence of bowel cancer. Eventually, he realized the more bulky, fiber-rich foods people eat, the less unhealthy fat they consume.

So chew a fiber-rich apple at every meal for a happy, healthy colon. You'll get the greatest nutritional value by eating an apple fresh and unpeeled. But it's a great food whether it's fresh from the tree or peeled, sliced, chopped, juiced, cooked, or sauced.

4 things you should know about apples

Here's how you can get the most benefits from this remarkable fruit.

You can check an apple's ripeness by its "under color" — the color of the peel in the core and stem cavities. For yellow or gold apples, the under color should be the same as the rest of the peel. In red varieties, look for green or yellow.

▶ *Buy apples that are unbruised,* firm, and have good color.

▶ *Store them loose in your refrigerator* in the produce bin or in a paper bag. Although they can be kept fresh a long time, studies show the antioxidants in the peel disappear rapidly in the first three months of cold storage.

▶ *Keep them away from strong-smelling foods,* like garlic and onions, because they will absorb odor.

▶ *Substitute applesauce for oil* or shortening in baked goods like muffins for fewer calories and extra moistness.

Artichokes
Ancient delicacy improves digestion

Artichokes have been cultivated, used as medicine, and enjoyed as a delicacy for thousands of years. Records show they were first grown in Ethiopia, then made their way to the Mediterranean region and Europe. In ancient times they were considered a delicacy, fit only for the nobility. But the ancients also discovered another use for this delicious plant — to help with digestion.

Healthy benefits

▶ Soothes indigestion

▶ Prevents constipation

▶ Improves irritable bowel syndrome symptoms

Artichokes are packed with vitamins, especially vitamin C and folate; minerals; and fiber, making them an important source of nutritional help for good digestion.

Prevents constipation. The fiber in artichokes may help prevent constipation-related troubles. A single medium artichoke has more than 6 grams of fiber while a half cup of artichoke hearts delivers 4 1/2 grams.

Tames indigestion. If you feel sick to your stomach, overly full, and have abdominal pain, you may be suffering from indigestion. But artichokes contain special substances called phytochemicals that help digestion run smoothly again. In fact, artichokes are phytochemical gold mines.

Phytochemicals are compounds in plants that help your body resist disease. Certain phytochemicals in the artichoke's leaves stimulate bile production that helps with the digestion of fat and cholesterol. Scientists have extracted these phytochemicals into an herbal remedy marketed as artichoke leaf extract (ALE).

Several studies showed dramatic improvements in people with indigestion after they were treated with artichoke leaf extract. It could be they experienced the same bile shortage that's been blamed for boosting cholesterol. After all, if the liver doesn't produce enough bile, food does not break down properly, which may cause stomach pain and indigestion.

Eases IBS symptoms. Artichoke leaf extract has been found to soothe irritable bowel syndrome (IBS) as well. A group of IBS sufferers were studied for six weeks while taking the herbal extract. All reported significant reductions in the severity of their symptoms. Plus, 96 percent rated the remedy as better than or equal to other therapies they had tried.

Although the scientific verdict on artichoke leaf extract is still pending, artichokes are considered to be a healthy food. If you've eaten an

Word to the wise

Stay away from artichoke leaf extract if you have gallstones or other gall bladder problems. Artichoke leaf stimulates contractions in the gallbladder, which may cause gallstones to move and block your ducts. It could also lead to a rupture. Play it safe and talk to your doctor first.

artichoke, you know it's an interesting experience. The "leaves" you peel away and eat are actually the bracts, or petals, of the flower bud. The fleshy bracts enclose and protect the heart. Eating artichokes requires some patience, but if you make the effort, you'll be rewarded with a delicious, healthful treat.

6 things you should know about artichokes

Thinking of entering the ranks of artichoke aficionados? Let these tips guide you from the grocery store to the dining table.

▸ *Learn that quality is not based on size.* Artichoke size depends on where it grows on the stalk. Large ones come from the center; medium ones from side branches. The 2-ounce babies grow at the base.

▸ *Choose compact and heavy artichokes* with "scales" that are fleshy, thick, firm, and tightly closed. If they look dry or woody and have begun to spread apart, they're past their prime.

Nearly all artichokes grown commercially in the United States are grown in Monterey County, California. The heart of artichoke country is Castroville, which proudly declares itself to be "The Artichoke Center of the World." Even though California's artichoke yield is huge, Italy remains the number-one artichoke-growing nation, followed by Spain, France, Argentina, and Egypt.

▸ *Check for tiny holes in the stem.* They're a sign of worm damage. If you see them there, the damage is probably worse inside the bud.

▸ *Treat your artichokes with TLC.* They appear tough, but they're really tender. Refrigerate them in a plastic bag sprinkled with a few drops of water. They should last four or five days. Don't rinse, wash, cut, or trim them before storing them in the fridge.

▸ *Cook the whole artichoke* before you stuff it or prepare the heart. It will make your job easier.

▸ *Trim about a quarter inch* from each leaf. Then pull the leaves gently through your teeth to get at the soft velvety parts at the bottom.

Bananas
Perfect fruit soothes your stomach

Bananas are one of the most important food crops in the world. They have no fat, cholesterol, or sodium. And this popular snack is full of fiber, vitamin C, vitamin B6, folate, potassium, and complex carbohydrates. You can always find fresh bananas in the grocery store, and they taste great.

Often described as an ideal food, bananas originated in the Malaysian jungles thousands of years ago. Alexander the Great found them when he conquered India in 327 B.C., and they were brought to the Western hemisphere when Spanish explorers found the New World.

Healthy benefits

▶ Eases acid indigestion

▶ Neutralizes heartburn

▶ Helps stop diarrhea

Today, bananas are grown commercially in Latin and South America and parts of Africa. Refrigerated steamships made it possible to bring them to the United States for widespread distribution beginning in the late 1800s.

Douses heartburn and acid indigestion. A banana is simple to digest, which makes it easy on the stomach and a favorite food for babies and seniors. It's also a great remedy for heartburn and acid indigestion.

Ditches diarrhea. Eating bananas slows down the effects of diarrhea. A study in Bangladesh found that babies with diarrhea recovered quicker when fed a diet containing cooked green bananas. Green bananas are a variety of cooking bananas found in Africa and Asia. The researchers think pectin, a soluble fiber that firms your stool, is the reason these youngsters got better faster. The pectin and other fiber in regular bananas can help you ditch your own diarrhea, which hits average adults about four times a year.

Bananas are an important part of the BRAT diet for people recovering from diarrhea. This combination of Bananas, Rice, Applesauce, and Toast is rich in fiber and nutrition but gentle and bland enough to pass easily through a weakened digestive tract. An added benefit is the potassium in bananas. This mineral is one of the important electrolytes you lose during a bout of diarrhea.

Potassium replacement is just one reason bananas are also a great energy snack, especially for endurance athletes. Bananas have more digestible carbohydrates than any other fruit. Your body burns calories from carbs faster and easier than calories from protein or fat.

5 things you should know about bananas

Bananas are harvested and shipped every day of the year, so they are always in season. Here are a few tips to help you enjoy them more.

▸ *Be patient.* Bananas ripen best between 58 and 64 degrees Fahrenheit. They get mushy, split open, and lose their flavor if left in the sun too long. Even in tropical growing areas, bananas are harvested green and stored in moist, shady places to ripen slowly.

▸ *Choose wisely.* Bananas have seven stages of ripeness, but the last three stages are the most important for consumers. Bananas with green tips are best for cooking. Full-yellow fruit is best for eating, and yellow with brown spots is recommended for baking.

- *Grab an apple.* You can ripen bananas faster with an apple. Put them both in a brown paper bag out of the sunlight. Ethylene gas from the apple speeds up the maturing process.

- *Keep fully ripe bananas* in the refrigerator. Cool temperatures slow ripening. Their skin will turn black, but the fruit inside stays fresh.

- *Freeze overripe bananas.* Peel them and put them in a freezer bag. Eat them frozen for a sweet summer treat, or use them in baking or in frozen smoothies.

Bananas don't grow on trees. The banana plant is a giant herb from the same family as lilies, orchids, and palms. It grows from an underground stem, or rhizome, and is the largest plant on earth without a woody stem. Instead, its trunk is made up of overlapping leaves that wrap around each other to a height of 15 to 30 feet.

Beans
Live longer with amazing legumes

If you think beans are just a gas attack waiting to happen, then you don't know beans. These tasty legumes get a bad rap because of their well-known gassy side effects, but they actually have many good qualities that outweigh the bad.

High in protein and low in fat, beans pack a nutritious punch without laying on the calories. They also contain plenty of fiber, phytochemicals, and folate to keep you — and your digestive tract — in tip-top shape.

Healthy benefits

- Cures constipation
- Cuts odds of hemorrhoids
- Helps prevent diverticulosis
- Reduces colon cancer risk

Conquers constipation. Just one cup of cooked beans provides up to 15 grams of fiber. All that fiber helps keep your digestive system running smoothly, so you avoid constipation. As a result, you also prevent related conditions like hemorrhoids and diverticulosis.

Stands against colon cancer. Some people call beans "the poor man's meat" because they're such a cheap way to get protein. But you don't have to be poor — just smart — to swap beans for meat. Not only will you lower your cholesterol, you'll also lower your risk for colon cancer.

That's largely because of fiber and resistant starch, the kind your body can't digest. Both substances pass undigested through your stomach and small intestine. When they settle in your colon, bacteria attack it. That produces butyrate, a compound that helps prevent cancer. Folate also lessens your risk of cancer and is especially helpful for people with a history of colon cancer.

Like red meat? You can still lower cancer risks by adding beans to your plate. Research shows you can lower your risk for colon cancer, without giving up red meat, by eating legumes at least three times a week.

Word to the wise

Beware of cooking beans in crockpots that don't get hot enough to boil water. Some beans are actually toxic if they are heated to about 175 degrees, but not boiled.

Symptoms of poisoning include vomiting, diarrhea, and stomach pain within one to three hours after eating. Fortunately, most people recover within a day.

Beans come in several varieties, including kidney, Great Northern, pinto, navy, and lima. But which bean is tops for colon health? That honor goes to the black bean. Studies show black beans rank No. 1 in fiber, resistant starch, and flavonoids, which act as antioxidants to battle cancer.

Beans even provide flour power for people who have celiac disease. Instead of wheat flour, which contains gluten, use or look for products made with gluten-free whole-bean flour.

Need any more evidence of the benefit of beans? They can help you live longer. An Australian study found that for every 20-gram (about three-fourths of an ounce) increase of legumes to your daily diet, your risk of death drops 7 to 8 percent.

In addition to beans, legumes include peas, lentils, and soybeans.

2 things you should know about beans

Beans are very, very good for you. Economical, too. Now you can enjoy them without embarrassing side effects. You don't have to put up with intestinal gas if you follow these tips.

- ▶ *Prepare dried beans* by soaking the beans for four to five hours, then draining. Cover with fresh water and boil for 10 minutes. Simmer for 30 minutes. Drain and cover with more water. Simmer until the beans are tender, about one to two hours.

- ▶ *Try Beano,* a product to help cut down on gas. Just add a few drops to your cooked beans before eating.

Even the government realizes the benefits of beans. The new Dietary Guidelines for Americans, released in January 2005 by the Department of Health and Human Services and the USDA, encourage people to eat three cups of beans a week, based on a 2,000-calorie daily diet.

Blueberries
Say goodbye to digestive blues

North America is the blueberry's homeland. It grows on shrubs, and each delicious berry forms on the heels of a pretty five-pointed flower. For that reason, early native-Americans called them "star berries."

You can thank the Wampanoag Indians for introducing this native berry to the Pilgrims after their first winter in the New World. Since then, the blueberry's popularity has spread around the globe.

The United States and Canada lead the world's blueberry production, but South America, Europe, Australia, and New Zealand also cultivate it. Japan and Iceland are two of the blueberry-loving countries that import large quantities of this luscious fruit.

Healthy benefits

▶ Helps cure diarrhea

▶ Prevents constipation and irregularity

▶ Combats cancers of the esophagus, stomach, colon, and liver

Counteracts constipation. Blueberries definitely qualify as a "functional food." Their fiber and phytochemicals are the source of the berries' protective and curative powers. A single cup has 3.5 grams of fiber, about 15 percent of the daily recommended intake. This alone is a sure-fire remedy for irregularity and constipation.

Vanquishes diarrhea. Surprisingly, blueberries may also help prevent diarrhea. The people of Sweden have used dried blueberries for hundreds of years as a diarrhea cure. It could be blueberries counteract the bacteria causing the problem, or perhaps it's a result of their soluble fiber. However, eating excessive amounts of wild blueberries that contain lots of insoluble fiber could cause diarrhea, so go easy on this variety.

Fights colon cancer. Phytochemicals, which include antioxidants, are blueberries' powerful disease fighters. Researchers at the USDA Human Nutrition Center have found blueberries to be tops in antioxidants among 40 other fresh fruits and vegetables. Blueberries are chock full of potent phytochemicals like these.

▶ *Lutein* is linked to reduced risk of colon cancer.

▶ *Resveratrol* acts against linoleic acid, a fatty acid present in high amounts in typical Western diets, which promotes colon cancer. Eating food containing resveratrol appears to help block a wide range of cancers.

▸ **Piceatannol** may put the brakes on the growth of colon cancer cells.

▸ **Ellagic acid** is a proven anti-cancer chemical that zeroes in on esophageal and colon cancers. It triggers enzymes that make cancer-causing substances water soluble. Once this happens, they're easy for the body to expel.

Battles stomach and liver cancers. The blueberry even has phyto-chemical defenders for other digestive organs.

▸ **Proanthocyanidins** are a class of antioxidants that appear to pre-vent cancer cells from multiplying. A test tube study showed they inhibited the growth of stomach and other cancer cells by up to 73 percent.

▸ **Pterostilbene** may inhibit can-cer growth in the liver.

Blueberries pack a powerful punch, so find ways to add them to your diet. Toss some on your cereal, in your morning muffins or pancakes, or on your ice cream or yogurt, and enjoy.

Not only is the blueberry one of the few fruits native to North America, it's also one of the few truly blue foods on earth. Anthocyanin, the com-pound that gives a blueberry its deep blue color, is also one of its powerful, disease-preventing antioxidants.

4 things you should know about blueberries

Keeping a healthy stock of blueberries on hand is simple. Just follow these easy tips.

▸ **Buy them fresh if in season**, or frozen if not, for the same nutri-tional benefits.

▸ **Freeze what you can't eat** while they're fresh. But don't rinse them ahead of time. They'll end up in a big frozen block.

▸ **Pick the blueberries yourself.** That's possible if you live in one of the 38 states where blueberries are grown commercially. The Web site

Word to the wise

You may enjoy blueberries most in your favorite cobbler or pie. Unfortunately, heat destroys some of the blueberry's precious nutrients. To enjoy their maximum benefit, eat them uncooked.

www.nabcblues.org/upick.htm will help you locate U-pick farms near you.

▶ ***Read ingredient labels.*** Some blueberry products are made with "sugar-enriched" dehydrated blueberries. Insist on the real thing, and accept no substitutes.

Broccoli sprouts
Knock out risky bacteria with sprouts

They say youth is wasted on the young. But when it comes to broccoli, younger means better. Like child prodigies, broccoli sprouts demonstrate remarkable ability early in life. In fact, they're most potent when they're only three days old. These baby bloomers even outshine the grown-up version of broccoli in fighting cancer and gastrointestinal disorders.

Healthy benefits

▶ Helps fight ulcers

▶ Eases gastritis

▶ Trims stomach cancer risk

Everyone knows about the health benefits of broccoli, the green, crown-topped member of the Brassica family, which also includes cabbage, cauliflower, kale, and brussels sprouts. But broccoli sprouts are just starting to gain attention. And it's about time.

If you, like former U.S. President George H.W. Bush, can't stand broccoli, don't worry. Broccoli sprouts have a peppery flavor and taste more like mild radishes than broccoli.

Developed by Johns Hopkins researchers, these tiny powerhouses are sold under the name BroccoSprouts. Each batch meets strict safety standards, so you don't have to worry about *Salmonella* or *E. coli*. Look for them in your local supermarket or health food store.

What makes broccoli sprouts so mighty? They're loaded with the phytochemical sulforaphane, the substance that gives broccoli its power. Broccoli sprouts boast 20 to 50 times more sulforaphane than regular broccoli.

While sulforaphane is their main weapon, broccoli sprouts also contain plenty of vitamin C, fiber, and calcium, making them an all-around healthy food.

Attacks ulcers. In laboratories and human studies, broccoli sprouts have so far lived up to their lofty potential. The biggest, and most recent, discovery is sulforaphane's antibacterial powers. In laboratory tests, sulforaphane isolated from broccoli seeds wiped out *H. pylori*,

Maximize the power of broccoli

A new study suggests you could be getting less cancer protection from the sulforaphane in broccoli if you don't have GSTM1 — a gene that helps grab sulforaphane's cancer-fighting power. About 50 percent of the population doesn't have this gene. But scientists found that a new "super" broccoli, containing three times as much sulforaphane as regular broccoli, helped people without GSTM1 hang on to sulforaphane and its protection.

In related research studies, people who ate a diet high in Chinese cabbage, regular cabbage, and other cruciferous vegetables also got more cancer protection. This study was small and only examined the short-term effects of broccoli, so stay tuned to see if future research confirms these results. Meanwhile, keep eating plenty of cruciferous veggies, including broccoli sprouts, Chinese cabbage, broccoli, turnips, and turnip greens.

the bacteria responsible for ulcers, gastritis, and other stomach problems, including stomach cancer.

Sulforaphane did this much better than other previously tested natural compounds, including allicin from garlic and resveratrol from grape skins and red wine. It even worked against strains of H. *pylori* that were resistant to certain antibiotics.

This means broccoli sprouts may be a cheaper, safer, effective alternative or addition to antibiotic treatment to get rid of H. *pylori* infections, a common problem throughout the world.

Drives back gastritis. Two recent studies involving people with H. *pylori* infections showed just how effective broccoli sprouts might be.

In the latest study, 40 people were given 100 grams (or 3 1/2 ounces) of either broccoli sprouts or alfalfa sprouts — which are similar to broccoli sprouts except they have almost no sulforaphane — every day for two months. Broccoli sprouts stopped H. *pylori* from setting up colonies and reduced the symptoms of gastritis, while alfalfa sprouts did not.

Sulforaphane kills the H. *pylori* bacterium that hides in the stomach lining and causes gastritis and ulcers. Could sulforaphane also help combat other digestive disturbances, like Crohn's disease, that may be triggered by a different bacterium, *mycobacterium avium paratuberculosis* (MAP)? This is an interesting possibility, but watch out! This could cause problems because chunky cruciferous vegetables, like broccoli, cauliflower, and cabbage, may aggravate inflammatory bowel diseases, such as Crohn's or ulcerative colitis. However, it might be interesting to see if sulforaphane that has been added to products like Brassica teas

Brassica teas are patented and licensed by Johns Hopkins University. They are available in several varieties — green tea, black tea, and Red Bush tea. For more information, call toll-free at 877-747-1277 or visit www.brassica.com on the Internet.

might be helpful in killing bacteria that may cause other digestive diseases without irritating the inflamed areas.

Defends against cancer. Sulforaphane's reputation was built on its cancer-fighting powers. It belongs to a group of phytochemicals called isothiocyanates, which serve as indirect antioxidants.

Unlike more well-known antioxidants, such as vitamin C and vitamin E, sulforaphane acts indirectly. Instead of taking on harmful free radicals itself, sulforaphane spurs your body's phase 2 detoxification enzymes into action. This stimulates your immune system to fight off disease. Its effects also last longer than regular antioxidants.

These long-lasting effects mean you may only need to eat a half cup of broccoli sprouts every other day to reap their benefits. Sulforaphane's antibiotic benefits don't increase if a larger amount is consumed. Therefore, it's wise not to overdo a good thing. However, sulforaphane's presumed anti-cancer effects may be more dose-related than the antibiotic effects. The optimal amount for combating cancer is yet to be determined.

> One half-cup serving of BroccoSprouts has as much sulforaphane as 1 1/4 pounds of mature broccoli.

Studies done on rodents show sulforaphane blocks mammary, colon, and stomach tumors. In theory, it should work in humans, too, but so far there's no proof — other than the often-noted association that people who eat broccoli have much lower rates of many cancers. But be patient. Broccoli sprouts research is booming and more good news could be just around the corner.

"Research in this area has exploded — both in the United States and internationally," says Johns Hopkins researcher Jed W. Fahey, who is setting up a study in South America.

Keep an eye on broccoli sprouts. Unlike some child prodigies that burn out before adulthood, broccoli sprouts may prove even better as time goes by.

4 things you should know about broccoli sprouts

Keep broccoli sprouts refrigerated, and they should last a week or two beyond their "sell by" date. Not sure how to fit broccoli sprouts into your diet? Try these suggestions.

▸ **Use broccoli sprouts instead of lettuce** on sandwiches.

▸ **Add broccoli sprouts to salads** or soups.

▸ **Garnish chicken,** pasta, or fish with broccoli sprouts.

▸ **Surf the Web.** You can find all kinds of recipes for broccoli sprouts, including those for pizza, pasta, and wraps, at *www.broccosprouts.com.* Just click on the recipes link.

Play it safe when sprouting at home

As a daredevil might say before his next big stunt, "Don't try this at home." That might be sound advice when it comes to growing your own broccoli sprouts.

Word to the wise

Researchers have found that microwaving and good old-fashioned boiling leaches sulforaphane and health-building polyphenols out of broccoli and broccoli sprouts. But steaming hangs on to cancer-fighting nutrients. Stick with speedy cooking methods or cooking techniques that put the broccoli or sprouts in as little water as possible.

Food-borne illness from bacteria, like *Salmonella* and *E. coli,* has been a concern with sprouts, prompting the FDA to toughen its standards. However, not all companies follow the FDA's guidelines for sprout production.

Keep in mind that contamination can occur at any point during the seeds' journey from the fields to your kitchen. Whether from bad water or soil, improperly composted manure, farm animals, harvesting equipment, storage containers, or mills, seeds encounter many possible dangers.

Brassica Protection Products, the company that sells BroccoSprouts, uses patented technology and strict sanitation guidelines to ensure its sprouts and seeds are safe. You can sprout your own broccoli sprouts from seeds, which also contain high amounts of sulforaphane. (For more information about Brassica Protection Products, including BroccoSprouts and Brassica teas, visit their Web site at *www.brassica.com* or call toll-free 877-747-1277).

Make sure you take precautions to avoid contamination. First, buy your seeds from a reputable company. Your best bet is Caudill Seed Company, the only company that meets the tough standards set by Brassica Protection Products.

You can purchase seeds from Caudill Seed Company by calling toll-free 800-695-2241. Seeds cost $9.50 per pound. Shipping and handling is extra. Of course, you can buy from other seed companies. But you might have to take some extra steps, like soaking your seeds in hot water, to make sure they're not contaminated.

For detailed instructions from the Ohio State University extension service, go to *http://ohioline.osu.edu/hyg-fact/3000/3085.html*.

No matter where you get your seeds, always follow the sprouting directions carefully. Otherwise, like that crazy daredevil, you're walking a tightrope without a net.

Cabbage
Sauerkraut short-circuits colon problems

Cabbage is the head of a family of cruciferous vegetables well known for promoting good digestive health and protecting against colon cancer. But you can get even better cancer protection from cabbage if

Healthy benefits

▶ Wards off cancer

▶ Improves digestion

▶ Eases constipation

you turn it into sauerkraut. Eat cabbage and its relatives to keep your intestinal tract healthy.

Crushes cancer. During the pickling process that ferments white cabbage into sauerkraut, cabbage glucosinolates break down into potent cancer-fighting isothiocyanates. These phytochemicals are particularly effective against colon, liver, lung, and breast cancers. They work by getting rid of enzymes that activate cancer cells and by boosting enzymes that kill cancer cells.

Cabbage and its brassica buddies have long been known for their generous supply of vitamin C, beta-carotene, and lutein. Those and other antioxidants make cabbage a hard-hitting cancer-fighter even without the added punch it gets as sauerkraut. But the benefits of cabbage come from more than just its individual ingredients. You need the whole food. For example, studies show people who eat more cruciferous vegetables, like cabbage, have less risk of cancer.

Another food made from fermented cabbage is kimchi, one of Korea's favorite dishes. It's made from Chinese cabbage, garlic, chili peppers, radishes, and other assorted ingredients. Korean studies have shown that eating some kinds of kimchi protects against stomach cancer. But people who eat saltier varieties of kimchi or pair it with foods high in nitrates are actually more likely to get cancer. The studies concluded that too much salt and nitrates would overpower the good effects of the vegetables. For the most benefit, choose lower-sodium varieties.

Word to the wise

Cabbage, like broccoli and beans, may cause some gas and bloating if you're not used to eating it. So add it to your diet a little at a time. Start with shredded cabbage in your salad or, if raw cabbage seems to be a problem, try cooked cabbage instead.

Aids digestion. Kimchi also has lots of lactic acid, which makes it an excellent digestive aid. Fermentation adds lactic acid and other organic acids to sauerkraut, as well, which makes it easier to digest. You can eat it plain, in salads, or along with other foods.

Combats constipation. Cabbage also battles constipation and the problems that come with it, like hemorrhoids and diverticular disease. That's because it's a rich source of fiber that bulks up your bowel movements and brings about easy elimination.

5 things you should know about cabbage

You can eat cabbage a variety of ways — from raw in coleslaw to cooked or sautéed with your main meal. Here are some hints to make the most of every leaf.

▸ *Pick a firm, heavy head* when shopping for cabbage.

▸ *Eat cabbage raw* or only lightly cooked for the most cancer protection. You can also serve coleslaw to put more cabbage on the table. Slaw is an excellent salad and, since it can be prepared so many ways, it's ideal for adding variety to your menus. Make it with a vinaigrette dressing instead of mayonnaise. Cabbage is a healthy, low-fat food as long as you don't drown it with a fatty dressing.

The health benefits of sauerkraut have long been known. James Cook and other 18th-century sea captains fed it to the crews of their sailing ships to prevent scurvy. The fermented sauerkraut was a way to preserve cabbage, a good source of vitamin C, which prevents the deadly disease.

▸ *Cook cabbage by cutting the head* into quarters and then boiling it gently for about 15 minutes. You can also stir-fry it until tender.

▸ *Rinse and drain sauerkraut* before serving since pickling adds lots of salt.

▸ *Substitute red cabbage* for iceberg lettuce in sandwiches, salads, and tacos. Red cabbage, both fresh and pickled, seems to have the most antioxidant power of all the cabbages. You'll get more nutrition along with extra color.

Cayenne pepper
Hot pepper heats up digestion

You might expect a chili pepper to set your stomach ablaze, but as it turns out, this hot spice could cool down your tummy troubles. Known by various names such as African pepper, bird pepper, chili pepper, Hungarian, sweet, and zanzibar pepper, the fruit of the cayenne plant can work wonders for digestion.

Healthy benefits

▶ Eases indigestion

▶ Gets rid of gas

▶ Banishes bloating

▶ Soothes constipation

▶ Nixes nausea

▶ Stops stomach pain

▶ Ends ulcers

Cayenne is healthy for the same reason it's spicy. It contains capsaicin, a pungent chemical that makes your mouth feel like it's burning. Capsaicin stimulates the nerve endings in your mouth, which makes your brain think you're in pain.

Capsaicin does more than just heat up your meals. It also heats up the digestive process. Pep up your next meal with cayenne pepper to save yourself from these pesky problems.

Helps regulate bowel movements. Capsaicin gets the juices flowing and the muscles moving in your stomach to speed up digestion. It also increases blood flow to your digestive tract, making it easier for your body to absorb nutrients from your food. This stimulates appetite and helps cure constipation.

Lets the air out of gas. Because capsaicin encourages digestive enzymes to flow through your intestines, food doesn't sit in your gut undigested. Capsaicin also kills the bacteria that cause gas when they feed off undigested food. That's how cayenne reduces gas and bloating.

Ends indigestion. Cayenne pepper may also cool an upset stomach if you have trouble after eating. A study from Italy showed that people who took red pepper before meals suffered nearly two-thirds less nausea, bloating, and stomach pain. For the study, they used the capsule form of red pepper, but you can get the same effect by eating three spicy meals.

Soothes stomach pain. Capsaicin is responsible for cayenne's ability to relieve stomach pain. It sends out an overload of messages, which overwhelms the nerves so they can't communicate pain very well. The nerves react by dumping out all their neurotransmitters, chemicals the nerves need to send pain signals to the brain, leaving them unable to register pain at all. This action is called a counterirritant effect.

At the same time, capsaicin reduces the amount of substance P in your stomach. Substance P is a brain chemical that carries pain signals. With less of it in your stomach, even fewer nerve impulses make it to the brain, so you feel less pain.

Helps heal ulcers. Another reason your stomach will love cayenne is its tendency to improve gastric ulcers. Depending on the dose, it can even stop the growth of *H. pylori*, the bacterium that causes ulcers. Scientists think capsaicin heals by increasing the blood flow around the stomach as well as the flow of protective mucus across the ulcer, while also killing *H. pylori*.

Word to the wise

Be careful not to get too much of a good thing. A study at the University of Chile showed a connection between gallbladder cancer and a diet high in chili peppers. Patients who ate a lot of chili peppers but not much fruit were more likely to get the cancer. If you have a history of gallbladder trouble, eat cayenne in moderation as part of a balanced diet.

3 things you should know about cayenne pepper

If you're new to cayenne, try a little bit at first, and then gradually add more as you get used to it. You'll be a pepper pro in no time. Until then, follow these helpful tips.

Cayenne pepper helped a Hungarian scientist get a Nobel Prize. Dr. Albert Szent-Gyorgyi had tried for years to find a plentiful source of vitamin C when his wife made him dinner with a chili pepper one night. On a whim, he took the pepper to his lab and checked it for vitamin C. It had so much that he was able to study the vitamin's structure and was awarded the Nobel Prize for it in 1937.

▶ *Start with a few drops of hot sauce* mixed into your food twice a day. Work your way up to one teaspoon per meal. Use hot sauce made with pure cayenne or chili peppers so you know it has capsaicin.

▶ *Wash your hands* after cutting up chili peppers. You want to keep cayenne from getting in your eyes because it burns so badly.

▶ *Make red pepper tea* by steeping one-fourth of a teaspoon of cayenne pepper in a cup of hot water. Or take one to two cayenne gelatin capsules one to three times a day to get your dose of this fiery healer.

Chamomile
Ancient remedy soothes modern ills

Chamomile tea has been nursing medical problems for more than 2,000 years and still treats digestive ailments today.

The ancient Egyptians used this "new" cure-all for anxiety, insomnia, dizziness, laryngitis, and skin conditions. In fact, they considered it so miraculous they dedicated the plant to their gods. Well-to-do Egyptian women even applied crushed chamomile petals to their skin as a

Healthy benefits

▶ Dries up diarrhea

▶ Nixes nausea

▶ Soothes stomach cramps

▶ Eliminates gas

▶ Prevents ulcers

▶ Beats bloating

▶ Alleviates acid reflux

cosmetic. Today, women often use it to lighten their hair as an alternative to harsh dyes and bleaches.

This flowering plant is a member of the daisy family, but it smells like apples, so you'll find the essential oil in soaps, creams, detergents, shampoos, and perfumes. The types of chamomile available include German, Hungarian, Roman and English, but the German type is used most often for healing.

You can make chamomile tea by steeping the dried flowering heads in boiling water. The heads release a tiny amount of blue oil made up of healing chemicals. The active ingredients in these chemicals are flavonoids and essential oils, which experts believe reduce inflammation and encourage healing. Drink chamomile tea and you just may find soothing relief for a variety of digestive ills.

Calms digestive distress.
Flavonoids in particular may be responsible for the anti-anxiety and sedative effects that make chamomile tea such a popular bedtime drink. They affect the same receptors in the brain as prescription drugs like Valium. The best news — you'll feel relaxed right away without suffering the addictive side effects you might from a drug.

Since it's especially good for soothing anxiety, chamomile may ease the tensions and spasms that cause stomach cramps, gas, bloating, nausea, and indigestion. Specific elements in chamomile are what

Word to the wise

Avoid drinking chamomile tea if you're allergic to ragweed. According to Dr. Leonard Bielory, director of the Asthma and Allergy Research Center at the University of Medicine and Dentistry of New Jersey, some herbs and fruits are cousins to ragweed, containing what he calls common proteins.

Bielory says you may find yourself sneezing, coughing, and experiencing other allergic symptoms when you eat cantaloupe, honeydew melon, and bananas — or when you drink chamomile tea.

scientists call antispasmodics — meaning they reduce spasms in your gastrointestinal tract.

Axes ulcers. Up to 50 percent of the essential oil in chamomile is alpha-bisabolol, an alcohol-based component. And it's very good at multi-tasking. Besides reducing muscle spasms, research shows alpha-bisabolol fights certain types of peptic ulcers.

Soothes inflammation. Apigenin is the most abundant flavonoid in chamomile flower heads. Its anti-inflammatory properties help tame stomach acid reflux and may soothe inflamed membranes like the ones that line your stomach.

3 things you should know about chamomile

Put the lid on muscle spasms with chamomile tea. Brew it fresh three to four times a day to soothe cramps and digestive disorders.

> ▸ *You can find chamomile tea at the grocery store,* but for best results, use dried flower heads or buy extracts from reputable companies and natural-food stores.

> ▸ *Steep a tablespoon of dried flowers* in a cup of hot water for 10 to 15 minutes.

> ▸ *Don't get too much of a good thing.* Some experts say more than four cups a day of chamomile tea may slow you down too much.

Cinnamon
Spicy way to ease stomach troubles

Cinnamon isn't just for sweet buns anymore. This condiment is a powerful antiseptic that acts against infectious diseases. In traditional Greek and Indian medicine, cinnamon treats bloating, indigestion, nausea, gas, and gastrointestinal spasms. Its healing capabilities and sweet taste have made it a valuable spice for thousands of years.

Cinnamon comes from the inner bark of the *Cinnamomum zeylanicum* tree. After the bark is removed, it's rolled into sticks. The sticks are then dried to use as is or ground into powder. The cinnamon from the C. *zeylanicum* tree is called "true cinnamon." Common cinnamon, the kind used in the United States, comes from the C. *cassia* tree.

Healthy benefits

▶ Kills E. coli

▶ Eases indigestion

▶ Soothes stomach upset

▶ Gets rid of gas

▶ Relieves bloating

▶ Ditches diarrhea

Fights food poisoning. Cinnamon spice is nice, except to bacteria. It nips *E. coli* in the bud. *E. coli* is a dangerous bacterium that causes severe diarrhea and flu-like symptoms. It usually turns up in unpasteurized food and undercooked meat.

The tree's bark, leaves, and roots all produce essential oils. These essential oils contain a substance that kills germs, especially *E. coli*. Researchers added cinnamon to apple juice infected with a large sample of *E. coli*. After three days at room temperature, the cinnamon destroyed more than 99 percent of the bacteria.

Aids digestion. Adding cinnamon to your meal does more than kill bacteria. It also aids digestion and relieves discomfort from indigestion. Scientists don't know exactly what cinnamon does to help digestion, but they think it has something to do with the way the spice heats up your stomach.

Calms stomach upset. Cinnamon also relieves upset stomach, gas, and diarrhea. Its volatile oils break down the fats in your intestinal tract, and the essential oils stimulate movement in the tract. This double action gets your system back to normal and relieves the feeling of being bloated.

3 things you should know about cinnamon

Whether you grind it, cook it, or brew it, try cinnamon to treat a variety of digestive dilemmas and add zip to your meals.

Word to the wise

Chewing cinnamon gum or sucking on cinnamon candy can cause a burning sensation in your mouth and trigger sores or ulcers to form. If you experience a reaction like this, avoid cinnamon gum and candy.

▶ *Use ground cinnamon to spice up desserts* like apple cobbler and pumpkin pie, or vegetables like cooked carrots, winter squash, and sweet potatoes.

▶ *Put cinnamon sticks in hot cider,* coffee drinks, and juices.

▶ *Make a tea* by stirring one-half to three-quarters of a teaspoon of powdered cinnamon in a cup of boiling water. Up to three cups a day helps intestinal problems, like indigestion, gas, and bloating. But don't eat cinnamon oil. It can be toxic even in small amounts.

Coffee
Tasty brew guards against gallstones

Coffee creates discussion. Friendly visits take place over a cup of coffee, and debates go on forever about whether coffee is good for you or not. People also talk a lot about how to make this tempting brew taste even better.

Discussion about coffee's health effects usually revolves around caffeine, the most popular and widely consumed drug in the United States. Coffee is a principal source of caffeine, and you'll find endless pros and cons about what it does to your body.

Healthy benefits

▶ Guards against gallstones

▶ May shrink colon cancer risk

Depending on your gastrointestinal situation, coffee and its caffeine — or possibly even coffee without the caffeine — may or may not help you. Let's get the bad news out of the way first.

Among caffeine's negative effects are upset stomach and diarrhea. Caffeine also relaxes your lower esophageal sphincter and allows acid reflux. It can be an irritable bowel syndrome (IBS) trigger, and IBS sufferers are often advised to cut out coffee and other caffeine sources. Caffeine may also aggravate the symptoms of restless legs syndrome.

Takes aim against colon cancer. On the plus side, a recent German study supports coffee as a colon cancer fighter. Scientists have long thought coffee's high antioxidant content helped prevent cancer. This study identifies an antioxidant called methylpyridinium, which specifically helps enzymes that protect against colon cancer.

Word to the wise

Coffee is not a substitute for water. It's a diuretic, which makes you lose fluids faster than usual. If you drink a lot of coffee, you need to drink extra water to replace what you lose. A lack of fluid will bring on constipation and may worsen other symptoms of irritable bowel syndrome.

Methylpyridinium is found almost exclusively in coffee. It is formed when coffee beans are roasted, and appears in both caffeinated and decaffeinated coffee. Laboratory tests and follow-up experiments on rats show it is a highly active anti-cancer compound. Further studies are planned to determine its exact effect on humans.

Protects gallbladder. Studies show caffeinated coffee may protect your gallbladder. The Harvard Nurses' Health study found women coffee drinkers had 25 percent less gallbladder surgery. Another Harvard study showed that men who drank two to four cups of coffee per day had 40 to 45 percent less risk. Research has also suggested coffee may help prevent gallstones, and one study found coffee relieved symptoms in women who already had gallstones. Scientists suspect coffee may get the muscles in both the gallbladder and the large bowel to move more. It also may affect bile flow.

Experts don't advise drinking coffee just to avoid gallstones. But they believe you have some added protection if you're already a coffee

The diuretic effect of coffee could cut your chances for kidney stones by 10 percent. Kidney stones don't have as much time to develop when you urinate more often. Surprisingly, decaf coffee lowers your risk about the same as regular coffee, leading researchers to believe it's more than just caffeine at work.

drinker. The same goes for the other benefits of coffee. As long as you don't have more than a couple of cups a day, you can enjoy the advantages and perhaps avoid the drawbacks.

3 things you should know about coffee

More shoppers have begun to choose fresh-roasted coffee beans you can grind yourself over the traditional already-ground variety. Here are some tips for getting the most out of your beans.

▸ *Keep coffee in an airtight container.* It is generally best if used a few days after roasting, but full flavor will stay for 10 days or more if it is not exposed to air.

▸ *Don't store coffee in the refrigerator.* Just like baking soda, coffee absorbs odors and flavors from other food products. Freezing can also damage coffee and is not recommended unless you need to store it for more than two weeks.

▸ *Grind coffee for drip brewing* to a consistency of granulated sugar, and grind only the amount you need at the time. Once the beans are ground, their flavorful oils are exposed to the air and will begin to evaporate immediately, taking your flavor with them.

Cranberries
Stop ulcers with a tiny berry

This native North American fruit flourishes in the coastal bogs of the Carolinas and northward into Canada. Before Europeans set foot in North America, North American Indians used cranberries as food and medicine for the treatment of bladder and kidney diseases. In recent years, its health benefits have been explored and confirmed through scientific research.

Researchers found that cranberries have more antioxidant phenols than any of the other 19 most popular fruits in the American diet. These phenols trigger the production of enzymes that make cancer-causing substances water soluble and easily eliminated from the body. The greatest antioxidant content is found in pure cranberry juice, next are fresh and dried berries, and then cranberry sauce. Juice drinks and cocktails have the least.

Thwarts traveler's diarrhea and UTIs. Health experts have known for years that cranberries battle bacteria. Studies show they prevent *E. coli* bacteria from sticking to the inner surface of your stomach, intestines, and urinary tract. These dangerous bacteria are responsible for traveler's diarrhea and some urinary tract infections, so making things slippery for them might lend you some protection. What's more, a new study shows that eating cranberries helps prevent tooth decay by the same anti-stick effect.

Fends off ulcers. Now researchers say cranberry works against ulcer-causing *H. pylori* bacteria in your stomach. One glass of cranberry juice a day could be enough to flush the bacteria out of your stomach before they can dig in and wreak havoc.

If you want the berry's benefits without the tartness, try cranberry juice extract supplements. You'll find them at health food stores.

4 things you should know about cranberries

It's a shame to limit your enjoyment of cranberries to cranberry sauce on festive occasions. Here's how to enjoy them year round.

Word to the wise

Consider limiting or avoiding cranberries if you're taking the anticoagulant warfarin. The combination could cause a dangerous drug interaction. Also, if you take calcium supplements, the oxalates in cranberries can make it more difficult for your body to absorb the calcium.

People who have kidney or gallbladder problems should also beware. Cranberry oxalates may bind with calcium and form stones.

▸ *Add some zing to cereal* or fruit salad with dehydrated berries. Dried cranberries are sold in grocery stores everywhere. You'll find them with the other dried fruits.

▸ *Take advantage of their natural tartness.* Try cranberries as a substitute for lemon or vinegar when you're dressing salad greens.

▸ *Keep them fresh for about two months* in your refrigerator. When you take them out, they may look damp, but that's OK. Just cull out any bad berries.

▸ *Freeze them so you'll have some on hand* until next year's crop comes in. Spread them out on a cookie sheet and stick them in the freezer for several hours. Dump the frozen berries into a freezer bag and date the bag. Once you thaw them, the berries will be soft, so use them right away.

Dried plums
New twist on a legendary fruit

Prunes, a well-known remedy for constipation, have a new name and a new image. The California Dried Plum Board thought the name "prune" limited its product to hospital and nursing home menus. They wanted to tout this tasty, wrinkled morsel as more than just a laxative.

California growers, who produce virtually all the prunes eaten in the United States and a majority worldwide, have changed their marketing strategy. You'll find the words "dried plums" on their packages instead of "prunes." And their high-fiber content, vitamins, minerals, and antioxidants are now getting all the attention.

The antioxidants in dried plums can slow down the effects of aging on the gut. Typical ailments of the aging gut include ulcers, constipation, diverticulosis, acid reflux, gallstones, leaky gut, and cancer.

Healthy benefits
▶ Prevents and mends constipation
▶ Helps avert or stop diarrhea
▶ Stifles bacterial infections like *E. coli*

Damage from free radicals speeds up the aging process even more. Since antioxidants wipe out free radicals, you can keep your gut from getting old too fast by getting plenty of them in your diet. Dried plums are an incredible source of these life-lengthening antioxidants.

Researchers for the United States Department of Agriculture measure and study antioxidants in food. Although their latest study examined 100 more foods than earlier research projects, the dried plum still fought off the contenders and made the top 10 list of antioxidant-rich foods. What's more, the dried plum is still a digestive health hero.

Fights food poisoning. You can eat dried plums by themselves or add them to other food to make it taste better and keep it safe to eat. Studies have shown that prune puree will kill certain strains of bacteria that cause food poisoning. Just one tablespoon per pound of ground beef, for instance, will kill up to 90 percent of *E. coli*, but this may not be enough to completely protect against food poisoning.

Defeats constipation. Just because dried plums are becoming famous for their other qualities, don't think they are any less valuable for keeping you regular.

According to a University of California at Davis (UC Davis) study, men who ate 12 dried plums a day increased their stool volume by 20 percent. As an added bonus, they also lowered their cholesterol significantly. The researchers believed the high amount of fiber — about

Word to the wise

Don't dry plums yourself. Commercial dehydration preserves nutrition, but foods dried in heated ovens at home can have a drastic loss of nutrients. The removal of water in dried fruit concentrates nutrients and reduces weight and volume. It also eliminates spoilage from bacteria and other microbes, which need water to grow.

7 grams for 12 dried plums — is a key to both the laxative action and the cholesterol lowering.

But the laxative power of dried plums comes from more than just their insoluble fiber. Prune juice also acts as a laxative, but it doesn't have any fiber. It is unclear just where the extra push comes from, but two substances that probably contribute are phenolic compounds, which also slow down glucose absorption, and sorbitol, a natural sugar that can cause diarrhea if you get too much of it.

Prevents diarrhea. The UC Davis study had one surprising finding. Eating 12 dried plums daily did not cause diarrhea in the men who participated. That may have happened because fiber in dried plums is 60 percent pectin. This soluble fiber has a slightly congealing effect in your intestines, which helps firm things up to relieve, or prevent, diarrhea.

3 things you should know about dried plums

Dried plums make a great snack right out of the package, but they're also great to use in cooking and baking.

▸ *Substitute one-fourth cup* of dried plum puree and a half cup of oil when the recipe calls for a cup of oil or butter in cakes, muffins, cookies, or brownies. To make the puree, combine 1 1/3 cups of pitted dried plums and 6 tablespoons of hot water in a food processor, and puree. Store in your refrigerator for up to one month.

- **Mix in some dried plum puree** to make moister meatballs — even from ground turkey. A few spoonfuls per pound of turkey will do the trick.

- **Use chopped dried plums** instead of raisins in cookies and muffins, or add them to your favorite cereal.

Prune juice isn't juice at all. It's really pulverized dried plums added to hot water. Rich in iron and potassium, it retains much more of the whole fruit's nutrients than most other fruit juices.

Fennel
Spicy way to relieve gas

In 490 B.C., the Greeks won an important victory over the Persians at a battle in Marathon, which means "the place of fennel." Today, you can win the war against embarrassing gas and stomach discomfort with the seeds of the plant after which that famous battleground was named.

Many people enjoy two main edible varieties of fennel — Florence and common. Both are tasty, aromatic additions to salads, soups, and various entrees, but only common fennel has the chewable, brewable seeds that make for a healthier digestive tract.

The fennel plant has closely arranged stalks topped with feathery green leaves. Its blooms are clusters of tiny golden flowers, which become the plant's "fruit" or seeds. The plants thrive almost anywhere and enjoy a long lifespan.

Healthy benefits

- Helps control diarrhea
- Clobbers constipation
- Diminishes gas
- Tames heartburn
- Calms indigestion
- Soothes stomachache
- Helps foil colon cancer
- Relaxes stomach and intestinal cramps

Fennel's stalks, leaves, and seeds are all edible, but Florence fennel also has edible bulbs. The plant's flavor and fragrance, which is similar to licorice, is sometimes mistaken for anise.

Improves digestion. The entire plant, but especially the seeds, contains essential oils. Chewing the seeds or drinking fennel-seed tea after a meal releases a compound called terpenoid anethole. This compound relieves spasms in the stomach and intestinal muscles.

By relaxing the muscles of the stomach and stimulating the production of bile, fennel also helps relieve cramps, diarrhea, gas, heartburn, indigestion, and stomachache. What's more, the fennel bulb contains soluble fiber, which also helps control diarrhea.

Word to the wise

Fennel seeds are harmless when used for brewing tea or munching after meals if you don't exceed the recommended amount. But more concentrated doses of their essential oils are a different matter.

Professionals who use these oils in the food, flavor, and fragrance industries understand their potential dangers. Too much can cause skin irritation, vomiting, seizures, and serious respiratory problems. For your safety's sake, steer clear of the oils and stick with the plant's greens and seeds.

Attacks constipation and colon cancer. The terpenoid anethole compound in fennel seeds, as well as the insoluble fiber from fennel bulb, helps speed up digestion. This reduces the amount of time food stays in your digestive tract, which could help prevent constipation and lower your risk of colon cancer by quickly removing cancer-causing toxins from your colon.

6 things you should know about fennel

Fresh fennel is best, so try growing it at home. It thrives almost anywhere. Your own plants can supply you with a season of greens and an abundance of seeds.

- **Score the greatest benefits** from seeds. They are the best source of fennel's essential oils.

- **Brew a flavorful tea** by steeping a teaspoon of fennel seeds in a cup of boiled water for 10 to 15 minutes. Strain out the seeds and enjoy. For a stronger tea, crush the seeds first.

- **Buy seeds as fresh as possible** from natural food markets or health food stores. Fennel seeds sold at grocery stores have probably been on the shelf a long time.

Have you ever eaten at an Indian restaurant and noticed a bowl of seeds on your table? This was fennel. These "Indian after-dinner mints" can freshen your breath and settle your stomach if you've eaten too much of that great Indian cuisine.

- **Store dried fennel seeds** in an airtight container in a cool, dry location. They'll be fine for about six months. Storing fennel seeds in the refrigerator will help to keep them fresh even longer.

- **Use the stalks and bulbs** in your favorite recipes. They are tasty and aromatic and can be braised, steamed, and sautéed.

- **Improve your salad's taste,** aroma, and nutritional value by adding fennel greens.

Figs
Delightful way to get more fiber

Figs are actually flowers turned inward into themselves. The tiny seeds within them are the real fruit. They're the only fruit that fully ripens and semi-dries right on the tree.

Healthy benefits

- Beats constipation
- Fends off colon cancer

They were also one of the first cultivated fruits. Since dried figs are easy to preserve and transport without refrigeration, they've been popular for thousands of years. You'll find references to figs in ancient literature, and the fig is mentioned in the Bible more than any other fruit.

Figs favor a climate similar to that found around the Mediterranean Sea. They were probably first cultivated in Egypt and Arabia. The figs you will most likely find at the market or growing in your community are varieties with names like Mission, Calimyrna, Kadota, and Adriatic — each with its own distinctive color and flavor.

If you have the opportunity to pick figs from trees in your area, seize it. The season usually extends from June to October. The drawback is that fresh figs don't keep long, even when refrigerated.

Word to the wise

Figs can cause high blood pressure, headaches, and neck pain if you're taking a certain type of antidepressant called a monoamine oxidase (MAO) inhibitor. Certain liver enzymes usually destroy a substance in figs called tyramine. However, MAO inhibitors reduce these enzymes allowing tyramine to build up to dangerous levels in your body. See your doctor if you experience any of these symptoms.

If you can't find fresh figs, look for dried figs, available year-round. You might also enjoy canned figs or fig concentrate, a purée used to flavor ice cream and other desserts. And don't forget fig bars, the cookies that made figs famous.

Cures constipation. One of the fig's claims to fame is its fiber. Figs are a small but mighty fruit. Five figs, fresh or dried, give you a whopping 9 grams of fiber, more than a third of the daily-recommended amount. It has more fiber per serving than apples, dates, dried plums, and many other fruits — dried or fresh. That's why figs help prevent constipation.

Guards against colon cancer. All that fiber may also fend off colon cancer by speeding the removal of cancer-causing toxins from your colon. In addition, figs score high marks for phenols — antioxidants that make your digestive tract an unattractive place for cancer cells to grow and congregate. These fig phenols stir up more antioxidant activity than green tea.

5 things you should know about figs

This delicious fruit is packed with calcium. A one-quarter cup serving of figs has 53 milligrams (mg) of calcium. A medium-size banana has only 5 mg. Here are some easy ways to add figs to your day.

▶ **Keep them handy.** They're a convenient snack and a quick, healthy way to satisfy your sweet tooth.

▶ **Add a few sliced figs** to tossed green salads for a special touch of flavor, sweetness, and texture.

▶ **Replace butter and margarine** with pureed figs as a tasty topping for winter squash and sweet potatoes.

▶ **Adorn a bagel with a spread** made by blending figs with low-fat cottage cheese, ricotta, or cream cheese.

▶ **Sweeten your favorite** hot or cold breakfast cereal with chopped figs instead of sugar.

Figs contain an enzyme called ficin that helps break down food as it digests. It was once used as the main ingredient in Adolph's Meat Tenderizer.

Flaxseed
Fantastic seed attacks cancer

Linen and flaxseed both come from the flax plant. You can set your table with the former — but save room on your plate for plenty of the latter.

Healthy benefits

▶ Stops constipation

▶ Combats colon cancer

▶ Tames IBD

Word to the wise

As with all high-fiber foods, add flaxseed to your diet gradually over time to let your body adjust. Otherwise, it may cause gas and other digestive problems. Make sure you drink plenty of fluids, too.

Flaxseed contains alpha-linolenic acid, a short-chain omega-3 fatty acid that provides many, but not all, of the important benefits associated with consumption of long-chain omega-3 fatty acids found in fish oil. In fact, flaxseed is the best plant source of omega-3 fatty acids, which not only protect your heart and ease arthritis, but may also help soothe your gastrointestinal tract. It's also loaded with fiber. Be smart and include some flaxseed in your diet every day.

Gets bowels moving again. Packed with both soluble and insoluble fiber, flaxseed bulks up your stool for an easy ride through your system. It doesn't take much to do the trick. Put a stop to constipation with as little as one tablespoon a day of this mighty food.

KO's cancer. But flaxseed's most powerful weapons might be its cancer-fighting phytochemicals — phenolic acids, flavonoids, and lignans. Flax is the top source of a lignan called secoisolariciresinol diglycoside (SDG), which research shows inhibits the formation and growth of new tumors. When you eat flaxseed, you help guard against breast, prostate, and colon cancer, and possibly other cancers as well.

Tames IBD. Because of all the fish they eat, Eskimos rarely get inflammatory bowel disease. Fish oil capsules can also help an irritated bowel. Consider flaxseed oil as a mild-flavored addition to fish or fish oil in your diet.

3 things you should know about flaxseed

You can find flaxseed in most health food stores and some grocery stores, either whole, ground, or in the form of flaxseed oil. Here's how to make this tiny dynamo a big part of your healthy lifestyle.

▶ *Find ways to add flaxseed to your diet.* Whip it into smoothies. Mix ground flaxseed in your oatmeal, rice pilaf, applesauce, or yogurt. Sprinkle some into your salads, soups, cereals, and baked goods. The best source of flaxseed meal may be from Rexall Sundown, available at Walmart. It's vacuum sealed in an airtight, resealable bag to retard spoilage and oxidation of the omega-3 fatty acids.

▶ *Check the expiration date of flaxseed oil.* Store it in the refrigerator and use within two months. If it smells too fishy, it's probably gone bad and you shouldn't use it. Use flaxseed oil on salads and vegetables instead of butter.

▶ *Grind flaxseed in a coffee grinder* and use as needed to preserve freshness.

You can get omega-3s from flaxseed indirectly. Some farmers feed their hens flaxseed to boost the omega-3 content of their eggs. These enriched eggs have about 8 to 10 times more omega-3 than regular eggs. Look for "modified fat" eggs or ones labeled "omega-3 enriched."

Garlic
Powerful herb kills bacteria

Garlic is an incredible herb. Ancient Egyptian slaves ate garlic to keep up their strength while they built the pyramids, and when Tutankhamen's tomb was opened, archaeologists found garlic cloves inside.

Healthy benefits

▶ Wages war on diarrhea

▶ Helps heal stomach ulcers

▶ Crushes cancer

Egyptians weren't the only ones who appreciated this odiferous herb. Roman warriors and gladiators ate it before a battle to give them courage. People in India used garlic for medicine as early as the sixth

Many spices can help wipe out the bacteria and fungi that cause food poisoning. This explains why dishes from tropical countries, like Mexico and Thailand, which are loaded with spices, might help fight the foodborne and water-borne bacterial diseases that are prevalent there. No matter where you live, adding spices and condiments to your food may help save you from a bout of nausea and vomiting. Everyday flavor-savers like garlic, onion, allspice, and oregano tested best in a Cornell University study. According to the researchers, they killed 100 percent of all bacteria in an international survey of spices used in cooking.

century B.C. In traditional Chinese medicine, garlic is a tonic that improves digestion in older people.

That may not be far off. Scientific research shows eating garlic may help prevent these serious conditions.

Battles diarrhea and ulcers. When crushed, garlic produces a powerful chemical called allicin, similar to penicillin. Allicin breaks down into several sulfur compounds and a substance called ajoene, which give garlic its distinctive smell.

The allicin in garlic seems to be an all-purpose microbe killer. It can take on bacteria, viruses, molds, yeasts, and other parasites. A study done in China showed that garlic can even kill *E. coli*, a bacterium that causes severe diarrhea. The allicin in garlic kills four types of *H. pylori*, the bacteria behind nagging stomach ulcers.

Puts the squeeze on cancer. Garlic fights cancer, too. Researchers in China noticed that people who ate a lot of garlic were less likely to get cancer of the stomach and esophagus than people who didn't eat garlic. Other studies have also shown a connection between eating garlic and a lower risk of colon, prostate, bladder, skin, and lung cancers.

The sulfur compounds, flavonoids, and vitamin C in garlic are antioxidants, and they capture free radicals, which can cause cell damage. Allicin and its sulfur compounds also order more of your body's mighty immune cells into battle. These tiny soldiers kill tumors and cancer cells. Garlic even contains germanium and selenium, trace elements that fight tumors.

7 things you should know about garlic

Experts recommend eating from one-half to three cloves of garlic a day. You can also take garlic powder or garlic supplements. In Germany, garlic supplements are the best-selling, over-the-counter medicine in pharmacies. Here's how to get on board with this helpful herb.

Word to the wise

Eating garlic, even small amounts, can cause upset stomach, heartburn, and intestinal problems for some people. It also thins your blood, so talk with your doctor before eating garlic or taking supplements if you take blood-thinning medication.

- ▶ *Choose firm bulbs* with white, papery skin. Stay away from brown cloves.

- ▶ *Keep garlic in a cool, dry place* away from direct sunlight and humidity.

- ▶ *Don't store your garlic in plastic bags* or sealed containers. If you need something to put garlic in, cut off the legs of a pair of pantyhose. Drop a bulb into the toe and tie a knot above it. One at a time, drop the rest of the bulbs into the hose and tie a knot after each one. Whenever you need some garlic, just snip off a section.

- ▶ *Crush or mince garlic* to make the most of its active ingredients. Then wait 10 minutes before you cook it.

- ▶ *Cook your garlic lightly,* if at all, to reap all the health benefits it has to offer. Cooking garlic destroys allicin and its sulfur compounds.

- ▶ *Sock E. coli* by adding three to five teaspoons of garlic powder to two pounds of ground beef. It will help protect you from that dangerous bacterium.

- ▶ *Beat the stink of garlic breath* by taking deodorized garlic pills, but don't overdo it. Large amounts in the range of 900 to 1,200 milligrams a day can cause a garlicky odor.

Ginger
Multi-talented spice settles stomach

Ginger isn't just for cooking. Though a popular ingredient in Asian recipes for thousands of years, ginger has been an essential remedy for generations in homes that place a high value on natural good health.

Healthy benefits

▶ Relieves nausea

▶ Stops indigestion

▶ Quiets upset stomach

▶ Settles abdominal cramps

▶ Neutralizes heartburn

▶ Ends gas and bloating

Ginger is chock full of phytochemicals, nutrients that give fruits and vegetables their color, scent, and flavor. Many of those phytochemicals are antioxidants that fight cancer by helping your body capture and flush out cancer-causing free radicals. Ginger has one of the highest antioxidant counts of all plants, a good reason to make this pungent spice a regular part of your diet.

Quiets cramps. One of those antioxidants is curcumin, a potent inflammation fighter. Curcumin is so effective it can reduce pain from arthritis, headaches, and muscle aches. Sometimes it even works as well as aspirin and ibuprofen, which makes it a good remedy for abdominal cramps.

Ginger may also be just as effective as nonsteroidal anti-inflammatory drugs (NSAIDs) at treating problems like arthritis pain, but with fewer side effects. Since ginger thins your blood like NSAIDs, you should check with your doctor before taking them at the same time. Don't take herbal supplements at all if you're scheduled for surgery or have gallbladder disease. It could lead to complications.

Zaps heartburn, indigestion, bloating, and gas. That's because ginger aids digestion and stimulates appetite by increasing the flow of saliva and gastric juices. It helps speed up digestion when your stomach is full from a huge meal. So if your eyes are bigger than your stomach, you'll find relief with ginger after overeating.

This spice also helps relieve heartburn, bloating, indigestion, and gas. Ginger promotes digestion so well many experts recommend eating 2 to 4 grams of it every day. That amount is equal to 500 to 1,000 milligrams of ginger supplement or one chunk of ginger root.

When the ancient Greeks first received ginger from the East, they noticed these desirable side effects, so they ended every evening meal by eating ginger wrapped in bread. This practice caught on, and the Greeks' after-dinner treat became the first cookie — gingerbread.

Shuts down nausea. The Greeks weren't the only ones who appreciated ginger. Ancient Chinese sailors ate chunks of it when they went out to sea to keep from getting seasick. Today you can still neutralize stomach discomfort with this safe, natural herb.

If you are prone to motion sickness, take some ginger about a half hour before traveling. It works in your gastrointestinal tract to relax nerves and muscles, which calms the vomiting reflex and reduces nausea. In one test, ginger prevented motion sickness better than the drug Dramamine. And ginger won't make you drowsy like most over-the-counter drugs used to treat motion sickness.

To keep a supply on hand, try growing this useful herb yourself. Just slice off two inches of ginger root and make sure the piece you cut off has an eye like a potato. Plant the piece in a 4-inch pot with the cut side down. Put it about an inch below the soil, and place the pot in a sunny window. Keep it moist, and a little ginger plant should appear in about a month, and before long, the ginger root will produce many new shoots. Then you'll have all the ginger you need at your fingertips.

6 things you should know about ginger

▸ *Make ginger tea* by simmering three or four slices of fresh ginger root in a pint of hot water for 10 to 15 minutes.

In the Middle Ages, theologians thought so much of ginger that they believed it must have come from the Garden of Eden. Whether that's true or not, we know how it got to America. Ginger came to the New World when Spanish explorers brought it over from Europe. Their first stop was Jamaica, where ginger beer is still a popular drink.

▶ *Toss some ginger into a stir-fry,* marinade, stew, sauce, or salad for a tasty and healthful meal.

▶ *Add it to your diet a little at a time,* until you're used to it, to avoid irritating your mouth or stomach.

▶ *Look for ginger root with thick branches* and tight skin when you shop. Pass on any that are shriveled or cracked.

▶ *Eat two pieces of candied* or crystallized ginger about a half hour before getting aboard a plane, boat, or car to prevent motion sickness. Take one or two more every four hours as needed. You can find candied ginger at Oriental markets and in some grocery stores.

▶ *Take one or two 500-milligram capsules* of ginger supplement to head off a queasy stomach. Or drink naturally, not artificially, flavored ginger ale. Just keep this in mind — ginger is a mild stimulant, so be careful about taking it before bedtime to help avoid insomnia.

Honey
Sweet remedy cures constipation

Honey is more than just a natural sweetener and an excellent topping for pancakes and biscuits. It's also a medicine that goes back to the ancient Egyptians, whose medical texts mentioned honey as early as 2600 B.C.

Healthy benefits

▶ Relieves constipation

▶ Knocks out peptic ulcers

▶ Controls diarrhea

▶ Helps heal gastritis

King Solomon said in Proverbs, "Eat honey, my son, for it is good."

Today, it's a valuable food and folk remedy and is regaining status as a legitimate medicine. Modern science has identified powerful antibacterial and antioxidant properties in honey.

Cures constipation. Honey has laxative powers that, in some cases, make it a natural cure for constipation. Honey contains fructose and glucose, two natural sugars. Fructose isn't quickly absorbed, so it acts as a natural laxative in the digestive tract, regulating digestion. Honey has more fructose than it does glucose, making it a natural cure that's better than fiber for some people. Take a few tablespoons of honey to clear constipation. One or two tablespoons of honey in a glass of water is a common remedy for constipation in Greece. Research shows three tablespoons work even better.

Axes ulcers. Honey's germ-killing properties are also especially effective against *H. pylori* bacteria, which cause gastritis and almost all peptic ulcers. But honey can kill *H. pylori* before it has a chance to damage your stomach. Try spreading a tablespoon of honey on a piece of bread and eating it an hour before meals and again at bedtime.

Ditches diarrhea. Because it can kill some bacteria that even the most powerful antibiotics can't, honey could be the best medicine available for bacteria-caused diarrhea.

All honey is not the same, because bees gather different nectar depending on where they are located. Many health experts at one time touted a particular New Zealand honey as having the most antibacterial power, but studies have shown honey from other parts of the world is just as good.

Word to the wise

The same laxative powers that let honey relieve constipation may aggravate irritable bowel syndrome. If you can't absorb fructose properly, it can result in bloating, cramps, and diarrhea. Soft drinks have high levels of fructose, so if you drink a lot of them, beware of those possible side effects.

4 things you should know about honey

Honey from every area is different because of local weather, climate, and variety of flowers — but all honey has healthful benefits. Just remember it is a sugar. A spoonful of honey actually has more calories than a spoonful of granulated sugar.

▶ *Be picky.* Darker honeys and raw honeys tend to have a stronger taste and more antioxidant power. What's more, raw or unprocessed honey has more potent germ-fighting powers than honey that has been purified by heating and skimming off unwanted material. That's because heating also destroys most of its antibacterial power. Too much sunlight does the same thing.

▶ *Store at room temperature.* Cold temperatures in your refrigerator will crystallize honey. To fix, simply put the jar in a saucepan of water and heat on low until the crystals dissolve. It's best to keep honey at room temperature and away from sunlight.

▶ *Breathe easier.* Honey may help you build up immunity from hay fever caused by pollen in the air, but stick with locally produced honey. It contains the same kind of pollen you breathe.

▶ *Don't give it to a baby.* Honey, especially raw honey, can cause food poisoning in babies. Isolated spores of harmful bacteria can cause an infection in a baby that would never occur in an adult with a capable immune system. Adults with normal immune systems are protected, but you should never feed honey to infants less than one year of age.

For more information

The American Apitherapy Society has a wealth of information about using honey for health and nutrition. Check out its Web site at www.apitherapy.org, or write to them at:

American Apitherapy Society
5535 Balboa Blvd
Suite 225
Encino, CA 91316

Kiwi
Avoid constipation with kiwi

Yang tao was once a delicacy enjoyed in the courts of China's great Khans. After its discovery by Europeans, it was renamed Chinese gooseberry because its taste and color reminded them of the European gooseberry. Finally, in 1974, New Zealanders adopted the more-marketable trade name kiwifruit because the fruit looks like their own brown, fuzzy kiwi bird. After this stroke of genius, sales of kiwifruit took off. And that's what it's been called ever since — but it will answer to "kiwi."

Healthy benefit

▶ Curbs constipation

Kiwifruit's most recent honor came when it was given a new scientific name, *Actinidia deliciosa*. Taste it and see if you can figure out why it got that name. This jewel of the Orient has a flavor all its own — the taste of strawberries, bananas, and pineapple in one fruit.

Researchers at Rutgers University, after studying kiwifruit, say it's the most nutrient dense of the 27 most commonly eaten fruits. A one-cup serving has 5 grams of fiber. It also has 164 milligrams of vitamin C. That's more than the daily recommended dietary allowance for adults.

Defends against constipation. Kiwifruit is a great addition to your daily diet and a boon to your digestive health. Research shows that regular consumption of kiwifruit will help keep you regular. It contributes to a bulkier, softer stool, which means more frequent bowel movements.

Researchers say a number of kiwi's ingredients make it good for your digestive tract, but they are certain kiwifruit's fiber is the main mover and shaker when it comes to constipation relief.

8 things you should know about kiwi

You'll find the once-rare kiwifruit in most grocery stores year round. Here's how to make the most of this delicious fruit.

▶ *Choose kiwi when they're plump* and a little soft.

▶ *Ripen them at room temperature* if they're too firm. Speed up the process by leaving them in a paper bag with an apple for a day or two.

▶ *Keep them in the refrigerator* for up to two weeks. Putting them in a plastic bag will keep them moist.

▶ *Add kiwi slices to salads, cereals, and beverages.* Kiwi make a great garnish for meat dishes, pies, and cakes. Blend them for delicious, milk-free smoothies.

▶ *Scoop the emerald fruit right from the skin* with a spoon, or quarter and eat them like apples. They're great with or without the skin.

▶ *Tenderize meat with kiwi.* The fruit contains a protein-digesting enzyme called actinidin. Just rub the kiwi's juicy flesh over the meat, and let stand for 10 to 15 minutes before you cook it.

Word to the wise

Kiwifruit is an allergen for some people. If you're allergic to papayas or pineapples, it's possible you'll also be allergic to kiwifruit.

▶ *Heat kiwi a few minutes* before adding it to gelatin recipes. The heat deactivates the actinidin. Otherwise, the enzyme will keep gelatin from setting.

▶ *Use caution when you flavor dairy products* with kiwi. Actinidin also breaks down dairy proteins. If you mix kiwi with ice cream, yogurt, or sour cream, eat it right away.

Nuts
Crack a snack to combat gallstones

You don't have to be a Nutty Professor to learn to appreciate nuts. These shelled superheroes pack a big punch when it comes to your digestive health, even if they're not all technically nuts.

Some well-known nuts are not true nuts in the botanical sense, but they get grouped in the nut category for practical purposes. For example, almonds, cashews, and pine nuts are technically seeds, while peanuts belong to the legume family. Pretty nutty.

Whether you reach for walnuts, pecans, almonds, cashews, pine nuts, chestnuts, pistachios, hazelnuts, Brazils, Macadamias, or peanuts, you'll get more than a great snack — you'll also grab a handful of good health.

Nuts are good sources of protein, so they make a healthy alternative to meat. They also contain plenty of vitamin E and fiber. But most of their power comes from unsaturated fats.

Most nuts contain lots of monounsaturated fat, the kind that lowers bad cholesterol while boosting levels of good HDL cholesterol. Walnuts, which have been shown to lower bad LDL cholesterol, boast alpha-linolenic acid, a short-chain omega-3 polyunsaturated fatty acid similar to the longer-chain omega-3 fatty acids found in fish.

This popular snack, which can also help protect you from heart disease, may help prevent the following digestive conditions.

Guards against gallbladder problems. These fats may explain why nuts protect against gallstones and gallbladder disease. A recent

Word to the wise

Nuts have a downside — many people are allergic to them. Peanut allergy is the most common nut allergy, affecting more than 3 million people and often causing severe, even fatal, reactions. Because of a certain protein, walnuts also rank among the top sources of food allergy. If you're allergic to walnuts, you could experience respiratory problems and stomach or skin irritation. If you discover you're allergic to peanuts or other nuts, protect yourself by becoming a conscientious label reader. Even a small amount of peanut or peanut oil can cause a serious reaction in sensitive people.

Harvard study showed that women who ate the most peanuts and other nuts had a 25-percent lower risk of cholecystectomy (surgical removal of the gallbladder) than women who never or rarely ate nuts.

Researchers speculate that, in addition to the fatty acids in nuts, other components, such as fiber, phytosterols, and magnesium, could contribute to the reduced risk of developing gallstones.

Crushes cancer. Nuts may also help prevent certain cancers, including colon cancer. Peanuts and other legumes contain beta-sitosterol, one of the estrogen-like plant compounds called phytosterols that may protect you from colon, breast, ovarian, and prostate cancers. Walnuts are one of the richest natural sources of ellagic acid, a flavonoid that fights cancerous tumors.

So crack open some nuts — and crack down on disease.

3 things you should know about nuts

Although nuts are a healthy choice, remember they are high in fat. An ounce of nuts has 13 to 20 grams of fat and 160 to 200 calories. It's still a good idea to add nuts to your diet, but don't go "nuts" over them.

▶ *Use nuts for baking or cooking,* add them to salads for crunch, or just eat a handful as a snack.

- *Nuts also make healthy oils.* Cook with peanut oil, a staple of Asian cooking, or walnut oil, which is great for salad dressings, baking, and sautéing.

- *Peanuts have many health benefits,* but they may be pro-inflammatory if eaten a lot because they are high in omega-6 fatty acids. The red skin of the peanut may also provoke a violent, life-threatening allergic reaction in some sensitive people. Go easy on peanuts, and balance their consumption with a variety of other nuts, like walnuts, that generally contain oils with anti-inflammatory properties.

Oats
Optimize health with an old-fashioned grain

You've heard the expression "healthy as a horse." And you probably know horses often eat oats. Coincidence? Doubtful.

Healthy benefits

- Protects against colon cancer
- Deters constipation

Oats, packed with fiber, protein, and key minerals, pull off a digestive Triple Crown — they help ease constipation, prevent colon cancer, and maintain a healthy gut.

You don't have to strap on a feedbag, but you might want to gallop to the grocery store for some of this healthy grain. Most oats you can buy are some form of oat groats, which are formed by removing the outer layer, toasting, and cleaning the oat. Rolled oats, or old-fashioned oats, are simply oat groats that have been steamed and flattened.

Other varieties include Scotch oats, steel-cut oats, or Irish oatmeal, which are all names for oats that have been cut but not rolled. You can also buy oat bran or oat flour. If you can't find these products in your supermarket, try a health food store.

Word to the wise

People with celiac disease are often told to avoid oats, along with wheat, rye, and barley, because of gluten. But recent Swedish studies show that adults with celiac disease can tolerate oats. However, some concern remains that people with this condition may experience abdominal discomfort and bloating. Talk with your doctor before adding oats to a gluten-free diet.

Wards off colon cancer. Oats' claim to fame rests with beta-glucan, a sticky type of soluble fiber. Beta-glucan slows food as it passes through your stomach and small intestine. This helps lower cholesterol and slows the absorption of carbohydrates, which keeps blood sugar under control.

But beta-glucan also speeds food through your large intestine, lowering your risk of colon cancer. It may also react with tiny organisms to form compounds that protect the colon wall and tame cancer-causing substances.

Repels constipation. The fiber in oats also keeps your digestive system running smoothly and prevents constipation. Remember, fiber acts as a natural laxative. It helps your colon form stools soft enough to pass quickly and easily through your system. Just make sure to drink plenty of water when you add fiber to your diet.

When it comes to fighting disease and maintaining a healthy gut, all it takes is some oats — and some good old-fashioned horse sense.

3 things you should know about oats

Oats are not just for horses. Find ways to fit more of this healthy grain into your diet.

▸ *Start your day with a bowl of oatmeal* or oat bran cereal. You can also sprinkle oat bran on your cereal or baked goods.

▸ *Cook oat groats as a side dish,* like rice, or use them in salads or stuffings.

▶ *Take your time.* While instant oatmeal may be quicker than cooking old-fashioned oats, remember it also contains added sugar and salt.

You can add oat bran to almost any recipe for bread, rolls, and biscuits, or you can buy bread made with oat bran at the store.

Olive oil
Change your oil to boost your health

Popeye and Bluto constantly fought over Olive Oyl in the cartoons. In real life, olive oil has health benefits worth fighting for.

Healthy benefits

▶ Cuts colon cancer risk

▶ Combats constipation

This flavorful oil, made by pressing ripe olives, has been a staple of the healthful Mediterranean diet for centuries. Rich in monounsaturated fat, vitamin E, and antioxidants, olive oil provides plenty of protection from disease.

While best known for its ability to lower cholesterol and blood pressure, olive oil does more than help your heart. It also fights diabetes and rheumatoid arthritis and may help you lose weight by making you feel full so you don't overeat.

Olive oil is no slouch when it comes to digestive problems, either. It may help prevent constipation and colon cancer.

Snubs colon cancer. Most of olive oil's power stems from its high monounsaturated fat content. In fact, with 77 percent oleic acid, a type of monounsaturated fat, olive oil boasts the highest proportion of monounsaturated fat of any oil.

Olive oil is not a new miracle cure. It's been around and prized for both cooking and healing for thousands of years. The Cretes grew rich from exporting olive oil as far back as 2475 B.C., and both the Bible and Greek mythology refer to it.

Monounsaturated fat cuts down on bad cholesterol without harming the good. But the oleic acid in olive oil may also help prevent colon cancer.

In laboratory tests, Spanish scientists found that both olive oil and oleic acid induce apoptosis, or cell death, in certain types of colon cancer cells. However, olive oil and oleic acid worked in different ways against another type of colon cancer cell, leading the researchers to conclude that other substances in olive oil also contribute to its cancer-fighting potential.

That's where vitamin E and other antioxidant compounds come in. They counteract harmful free radicals and may play an important role in preventing not only colon cancer, but also cancer of the breast, prostate, and esophagus.

Several studies, including a British study of the dietary patterns of people living in 28 countries, showed that adding olive oil to your diet might reduce the risk of colon cancer.

Thwarts constipation. Olive oil also works as a mild laxative. So if you're feeling constipated, you might just need a quick oil change.

3 things you should know about olive oil

Olive oil has been used for centuries to treat wounds, minor burns, eczema, and psoriasis. But it's still most effective as a food.

▶ *Look for "extra virgin" olive oil* for the most benefit. That's because it's the least refined and has the most beneficial substances. It also has the strongest flavor.

▶ *Keep olive oil away from heat and light* in a tightly closed container, and it can last up to two years. If you refrigerate it, it will become cloudy until it reaches room temperature again.

▶ **Substitute olive oil for butter,** margarine, or other vegetable oils when you cook. Because this tempting oil has so much flavor, you can use 25 percent less than the recipe calls for. It's also great for salad dressings and marinades.

Word to the wise

While olive oil is chock-full of benefits, it's also high in calories. Like most oils, it contains about 120 calories per tablespoon. So don't go overboard.

Onions
Put the bite on cancer

Onions are precious. At least, the Romans thought so. The English word *onion* came from their word *unio* — "large pearl."

Healthy benefits

▶ Cuts colon cancer risk

▶ Thwarts esophageal cancer

▶ Quells stomach cancer

▶ Helps heal ulcers

Onions are members of the allium family. Their cousins include garlic, chives, leeks, and shallots. Eat them raw in salads or on your favorite sandwich, and try them boiled or baked. Cooking calms their flavor and fragrance.

One of the best-selling vegetable crops in the world, onions are a mainstay in the diet of almost every culture. People everywhere love them because they enhance the flavor of everything.

These pungent vegetables are a little different from most garden produce. They don't require much care. They're tough, easily stored, and don't require refrigeration until they've been sliced and diced. The part most people eat is the fleshy, layered bulb. It's wrapped in a papery, protective skin and comes in a variety of colors, flavors, and strengths.

Onions are exceptionally rich in two kinds of antioxidants — anthocyanins and flavanols. They give onions their color. Anthocyanins make red onions red and purple onions purple. They're also responsible for the blues and reds of blueberries and raspberries.

The flavanol quercetin gives yellow and brown onions their golden hue. Tea, apples, and onions are all loaded with quercetin. But researchers have found that your body absorbs this antioxidant much better from onions than it can from tea or apples.

Onions get their full flavor and fragrance from another type of antioxidant called alkenyl cysteine sulphoxides — ACSOs, for short.

While digging around the onion bed, researchers discovered that the strong varieties of onions, like Western Yellow, New York Bold, and Northern Red, have lots of antioxidant activity. Much more, in fact, than the milder, sweeter varieties, like Vidalia. These great antioxidants do more than give onions their color, flavor, and fragrance. They also do your digestive tract some big favors.

Word to the wise

You just ate a big slice of onion, but you don't want everyone to know. Obliterate telltale "onion breath" by rinsing your mouth with lemon water, chewing a citrus peel, or eating a sprig of parsley.

Cuts your risk of cancer. Onions may reduce your risk of cancer, especially of the esophagus and stomach, and they can prevent the growth of cancer cells in your colon.

Puts a stop to ulcers. Onions' antioxidants also help stop gastric ulcers by scavenging for harmful free radicals and may even help stop the spread of the ulcer-causing bacteria H. pylori.

5 things you should know about onions

What variety — everything from pungent and tangy tear-jerkers to sweet eye-pleasers, from pearly whites to deep purples. Here is how you can make the most of this incredible vegetable.

▶ *Buy fresh onions of any variety* from March through August. These onions are thin-skinned and usually sweeter and milder than the varieties you'll find August through April, called "storage" onions.

▶ *Storage onions have thick, papery skins* that contain more of the antioxidant quercetin than the rest of the onion. Unfortunately, the skins are not edible. To reap the benefits, add the skins to soups and stews. Just remove them at the end of cooking like you would a bay leaf.

Every onion cell has two sections, each with its own chemicals. When sliced, the cells break open and their contents mix. This creates a gas which, when it reaches your eyes, reacts with your tears and forms sulfuric acid. That's what makes them sting and water.

▶ *Prevent onions from making you cry.* Cut them from the top down, and wait until the last moment to trim off the bottom end. The compound that makes your tears flow is concentrated there. Or try this — slice them under water. If that's impractical, just wet your hands and the onions before slicing.

▶ *Know the measure of an onion* — one medium bulb equals one cup of chopped onions.

▶ *Store onions in a cool, dry place* for up to two months.

Oregano
Potent spice a powerful healer

One of the most powerful healing herbs may already be in your spice rack. Oregano, a spice you've probably had in Italian food, is the leaves of the herb *Origanum vulgare.* This

Healthy benefits

▶ Protects against cancer

▶ Kills bacteria, parasites, fungi

▶ Soothes intestinal spasms

herb grows in the Mediterranean region and in Asia, and it's usually harvested in the wild.

The ancient Greeks and Egyptians used oregano to flavor vegetables, wines, meats, and fish. The Greeks must have valued the herb because the word "oregano" is Greek for "Joy of the Mountain."

But this savory spice does more than tickle your taste buds. If you want to keep the doctor away, a sprinkle of oregano a day beats an apple. In fact, a tablespoon ought to do the trick. Studies show one tablespoon of fresh oregano has as many antioxidants as an entire apple.

The U.S. Department of Agriculture compared 39 different herbs to find out which ones had the most antioxidants. Out of 27 herbs used for cooking and 12 used for medicine, the herbs with the highest counts were in the oregano family. Mexican, Italian, and Greek oregano all tested high in antioxidants.

In fact, oregano had 3 to 20 times more antioxidants than the other herbs. Ounce for ounce, it has 42 times the healing power of an apple, 30 times more than a potato, and 12 times more than an orange.

Word to the wise

Many herbs cause allergic reactions. Oregano sometimes causes a rash when it comes in contact with skin. Some people also have a reaction when they eat it. One 45-year-old woman was so allergic that she broke out in a rash only 20 minutes after eating the spice.

Fights cancer. Antioxidants destroy free radicals, which can damage your body's cells and lead to cancer. Oregano's antioxidant trio — thymol, carvacrol, and tocopherols — make it a heavyweight winner in the fight against free radicals.

Kills intestinal invaders. Thymol and carvacrol can destroy more than free radicals. Studies show that oregano and its essential oils can kill or prevent the growth of bacteria, including *Listeria, Pseudomonas, Proteus, Salmonella*, and *Clostridium*. It can also take on fungi.

Oregano even kills parasites. In one study, 14 people infected with parasites took oregano oil for six weeks. The oil killed parasites including *Endolimax nana, Entamoeba hartmanni,* and *Blastocystis hominis* in 13 study participants. Microbes like these can cause infections leading to diarrhea and other intestinal problems, so sprinkle on the oregano to protect yourself from illness.

Between the years 1948 and 1956, sales of oregano in the United States jumped 5,200 percent. The phenomenal boost was a result of the sudden demand for pizza and other Italian dishes servicemen had discovered in Europe during World War II.

Soothes intestinal spasms. In Morocco, they've found yet another use for oregano. People there make the leaves and flowers of oregano into a tea, which they drink to relieve intestinal spasms.

Tests show that the thymol and carvacrol in *Origanum compactum* can rapidly stabilize spasms. Your muscles need calcium to move. Experts think *O. compactum* blocks calcium from entering the membrane of the muscles. Without calcium, your muscles stop contracting, and you feel relief.

4 things you should know about oregano

Oregano makes a delicious and healthful addition to your favorite meals. Follow these suggestions to get every possible benefit from your dining experience.

▶ *Use fresh herbs* instead of dried. They have more antioxidants.

▶ *Add oregano at the beginning* of the cooking process, so the flavor has time to develop.

▶ *Toss it into salads,* add to dressings, sprinkle on pizza, or stir into soup and tomato sauce.

▶ *Be creative* — season lamb, poultry, shrimp, mushrooms, green beans, and squash.

Organic foods
Stay healthy with natural foods

Walk into any supermarket, and you'll see organic foods in the produce department, the dairy section, even the meat department. These foods are often touted as a healthier alternative to regular products, but their prices make them seem more like a gourmet treat.

Healthy benefits

▶ Curbs risk of colon cancer

▶ Stifles stomach cancer risk

▶ Helps prevent ulcers

So is it worth the extra dollars to put pesticide-free food on your table? Pesticides keep weeds, fungus, insects, and other predators away. That may sound like a good thing, but it keeps plants from drawing on their "inner resources" for protection. When plants have to fight off pests on their own, their astonishing immune system goes to work, producing extra phytochemicals to protect themselves. These high-powered nutrients are one reason fruits and veggies are so good for you.

The U.S. Department of Agriculture (USDA) recently implemented guidelines, standards, and definitions about "organically" grown foods to help you decide what to buy.

The USDA has monitored the use of pesticides, hormones, and irradiation for years. But now it has actually defined terms like "organic" and "organically grown." It requires any food labeled with those terms to measure up to rigorous standards the public can understand.

Now that such standards are available, researchers can compare the actual nutritional content of foods grown normally with those grown organically.

▶ One study discovered that organically grown corn, strawberries, and marionberries (a type of blackberry) have significantly more anti-cancer antioxidants than those grown using pesticides and herbicides.

▸ Another study by researchers in Scotland found that soups made of organic vegetables had six times more salicylic acid, a substance known to combat colon cancer, than nonorganic vegetables.

▸ A researcher at Johns Hopkins University learned that organically grown fruits and vegetables were higher in most vitamins and minerals and lower in certain potentially harmful chemicals.

A food won't necessarily make you healthier simply because it's organic. When it comes to what you eat and drink, take this approach when you shop. Mentally erase the word organic from the label. It may say "organic candy," but just think "candy." Would you still buy it without the organic label? If not, then don't.

The organic foods she examined had 29 percent more magnesium and 27 percent more vitamin C, nutrients important to digestive health. The tested organic crops also had 15 percent fewer nitrates, chemicals that increase the risk of stomach cancer, than foods grown conventionally.

These studies show that higher levels of antioxidants and other phytochemicals in organic foods can benefit your digestive tract in several ways.

Reduces risk of colon cancer. Salicylic acid is a close cousin to acetylsalicylic acid, which makes aspirin a potent anti-inflammatory medicine. Higher levels of salicylic acid in organically grown foods appear to help combat colon cancer. Magnesium, a mineral found in much higher concentrations in organic foods, may also reduce your risk of colon cancer.

Hammers *H. pylori*. Vitamin C may play a powerful role in preventing ulcers and stomach cancer caused by the bacterium *H. pylori*. Organically grown fruits and vegetables typically have high levels of vitamin C.

Preliminary findings indicate organic foods do provide a nutritional boost. It's up to you to decide if these products are worth the extra cost.

4 things you should know about organic foods

Thanks to USDA guidelines for food labeling, it's easier than ever to spot which foods are organic and which aren't.

▶ *Look for a label* that says "100 percent organic" if you want a "pure" product. That means no synthetic pesticides, herbicides, chemical fertilizers, antibiotics, hormones, additives, or preservatives have been used in the product's growth and preparation.

▶ *Understand that an "organic" label* means the product's ingredients are not totally pure but are at least 95-percent organic.

▶ *Watch for the phrase* "made with organic ingredients." This means only 70 percent of the product is organic.

▶ *Be on the lookout* for the word "organic" in ingredient lists. That means the food itself is less than 70 percent organic, but at least one of the ingredients is. Although the word can't appear on the front of the package, it can still be used if it only appears in the list of ingredients.

Papayas
Juicy fruit boosts stomach health

The papaya may not be the best-known item in the produce department, but it's a tasty tropical fruit that's also good for your stomach. Its many healthful ingredients help your digestion and may guard against colon cancer.

Healthy benefits

▶ Eases digestion

▶ Soothes IBS symptoms

▶ Guards against colon cancer

Calms digestion. One of those is papain, a unique enzyme that breaks down protein. It is abundant in unripe papayas but fades away as the fruit matures. Once the papaya ripens, only small amounts of the enzyme are left. When the fruit is ready to eat, it has just enough papain to gently boost your digestive process. You should cook unripe papayas before eating to lessen the effects of the enzyme.

Papain is extracted from unripe papayas as a milky latex, dried and used as an ingredient in meat tenderizers, among other things. In very low doses, it's also used as a digestive aid. Large amounts of this enzyme have been known to eat through the esophagus. The latex may cause severe gastritis in people who are allergic to it, and it can induce uterine contractions in pregnant women.

Fights colon cancer. Papayas also supply a rich source of fiber and several vitamins that cut your risk for many kinds of cancer, particularly colon cancer. One half of a papaya has more vitamin C than an orange. And it has folate, beta-carotene, and vitamin E, too.

Lycopene, another cancer-fighting antioxidant, is abundant in papayas. Most lycopene in Western diets comes from citrus and tomatoes, but if you can't handle the acid, tropical fruits like papayas and guava can provide protective lycopene without hurting your stomach.

Word to the wise

The papain in papaya may increase the effects of the drug warfarin. If you take a blood thinner or anything else that has warfarin in it, talk to your doctor before eating this fruit.

Controls IBS. If you suffer from irritable bowel syndrome, you may want to add papayas to your diet as well. The fiber and papain in papayas can help soothe your uncomfortable symptoms.

3 things you should know about papayas

This fruit's many varieties fall into two main types — Hawaiian and Mexican. Hawaiian papayas are pear-shaped, weigh about a pound each, and are usually sweeter. Mexican papayas are larger and can weigh up to 20 pounds. Here are some tips for enjoying this luscious fruit.

You cannot eat the peel of a papaya, but you can eat the small, black seeds in the middle of the fruit. Don't expect them to taste sweet, though. They are slightly bitter, similar to black pepper. You can sprinkle them in salads, or grind them in a pepper mill to use as seasoning.

▶ **Squeeze a papaya gently to see if it's ripe.** If it gives slightly but is not soft at the ends, it's just right. Depending on the variety, ripe papayas are partly to completely yellow in color. Avoid fruit with black spots or damage to the skin.

▶ **Eat a ripe papaya like a melon** by slicing it in half and scooping out the seeds. You can also cut it up and use it in fruit salads.

▶ **Cook unripe papayas the same as winter squash.** Look for other recipes for cooking both the ripe and unripe fruit.

Parsley
Hidden virtues of popular herb

Many people know parsley only as a frilly sprig of green that comes with a fancy restaurant meal. But others are convinced this herb has many healing powers.

Parsley is packed with vitamins, minerals, and cancer-fighting flavonoids. It's especially high in vitamin C, vitamin K, and iron.

Over the centuries, people have used parsley to cure a variety of ills ranging from stomach problems to baldness. One legend from the

Healthy benefit

▶ Relieves gas

British Isles says ancient Anglo-Saxons even used parsley to mend skulls broken in combat.

Defeats gas. As a folk remedy, it has been used to aid digestion, relieve gas, and cure intestinal problems. It's also used to flush the urinary tract and prevent kidney stones, as well as ease kidney and bladder inflammation. As a diuretic, it can help treat urinary tract infections.

Despite its many uses and reputed cures, scientific research has only validated that:

> ▸ parsley is high in nutritional value.
>
> ▸ it works as a diuretic and for relieving gas.
>
> ▸ it can freshen your breath and is particularly effective against garlic.

You can find fresh parsley in the produce section of your grocery store, or you can buy the dried and crushed leaves and stems. The parsley fruit, sometimes incorrectly called seeds, contains a volatile oil that may be responsible for this herb's mild diuretic effect. However, this oil is poisonous in highly concentrated form.

Word to the wise

Don't overdo parsley if you're pregnant or have kidney trouble. Large doses of parsley supplements or extracts can lead to spasms in the bladder, intestines, or uterus. Other harmful side effects include bloody stools, urinary problems, and mucous membrane bleeding.

3 things you should know about parsley

Parsley is easy to find and even easier to prepare. Here's how you can reap the most benefits from this fragrant herb.

> ▸ *Look for two types* when you're shopping. Curly leaf parsley is best for garnishes. Flat leaf, or Italian, parsley has a stronger

taste and is used more for cooking. Make sure the cuttings have crisp, bright green leaves.

The ancient Greeks believed parsley was sacred. They didn't eat it but used it to make crowns for athletic victors and wreaths for tombs of the dead. The Romans began using parsley as a garnish, and it seems to have become a seasoning sometime during the Middle Ages.

▶ *Place the stems in a cup of water* and refrigerate them if you plan to use the herb soon. For longer storage, rinse and chop, then freeze in a plastic bag. Or place minced parsley in ice cube trays, cover with water, and freeze. You can add the cubes directly to soups or stews.

▶ *Use parsley for more than just decorating* your plate. Top off sandwiches, dress up salads, and use it to flavor stews and sauces. Just toss the parsley in at the end to keep its color and nutrients.

Peppermint
Common herb packs a healing punch

Peppermint may be the most effective herbal therapy for certain digestive problems. This herb offers more than just a refreshing fragrance. It might help take care of a host of digestive ailments.

The plant itself is a member of the mint family. It grows along stream banks and in wetlands and has purple and lilac flowers. There are many types of peppermint, but peppermint oil is made from white

Healthy benefits

▶ Quiets stomach pain

▶ Stops bloating

▶ Diminishes gas

▶ Quells nausea

▶ Relaxes IBS symptoms

▶ Fights indigestion

▶ Attacks gallstones

peppermint, which has light green leaves, and black peppermint, which has dark green leaves.

Using peppermint for healing purposes is nothing new. Its healing powers were first written about in 17th-century England, but early records show the Greek, Roman, and Egyptian civilizations used mint leaves in medicine. The Greeks and Romans also used them for temple rituals.

In the Middle Ages, Europeans would sprinkle dried mint leaves all around their homes and beds to keep pests away and mask odors. They still make a good alternative to mothballs. Today, peppermint is used in a variety of products like lotions, cosmetics, bath products, antacids, toothpaste, and mouthwash.

But the main benefit of peppermint is its ability to soothe your stomach.

Beats IBS symptoms. Menthol, the active ingredient in peppermint, not only kills some bacteria that cause diarrhea, but also relieves spasms in the muscles of the digestive tract. This makes it helpful for ailments like irritable bowel syndrome (IBS). Peppermint oil seems to block calcium from getting into muscle cells, so they stop contracting and calm down. That's how it relaxes the smooth muscles lining the intestines.

Banishes bloating and gas. If you suffer from bloating and gas, peppermint helps by stimulating digestion and fighting flatulence. It relieves intestinal gas by triggering the flow of bile to break down

Word to the wise

Peppermint isn't perfect. For some people, it causes heartburn. A valve at the bottom of your esophagus opens and closes to let food in and out. Peppermint sometimes relaxes this valve so it opens more than it should and lets stomach acid back into your esophagus. That reflux is heartburn. If you're susceptible to heartburn, take enteric-coated capsules with 0.2 milliliters of peppermint oil. Take one capsule 30 to 60 minutes before each meal to help ease intestinal problems. Enteric-coated capsules containing peppermint oil wait until they're past your stomach to dissolve, so your esophagus is safe.

fats, which reduces bloating, gas, and flatulence. Peppermint also helps you burp, which is another way to release gas.

Pounces on gallstones. Extra bile in your system is a good thing. Not only does it get rid of bloating and gas, it also may help break down gallstones. But if you have gallstones, you should talk with your doctor first before trying peppermint.

Lulls stomach pain and indigestion. Peppermint leaves, either chewed or steeped in hot water, will also relieve indigestion, as well as stomach pain from bloating, gas, or IBS.

Stills nausea. Peppermint's ability to soothe digestive tract muscles means it may also help relieve nausea. To brew peppermint tea, pour 5 ounces of hot water over two teaspoons of peppermint leaves. Let it steep for 10 minutes.

3 things you should know about peppermint

You can take advantage of peppermint's soothing qualities in a tea or as a supplement. Here's how to get the greatest benefits from this healing herb.

▸ *Pour one cup boiling water* over one or two tablespoons of peppermint tea leaves, depending on how strong you like it. Steep for five minutes. Have a cup of peppermint tea between meals, but don't drink more than four cups a day.

▸ *Don't try peppermint remedies* on children since the menthol scent is too strong for them and may do more harm than good.

▸ *Use it safely.* Menthol, the active ingredient in peppermint, can be fatal if you swallow it in its pure form, so always make sure it's diluted before you take it. Diluted or not, check with your doctor before using peppermint if you have liver disease, gallbladder disease, hiatal hernia, or heartburn from gastroesophageal reflux disease (GERD). Peppermint could aggravate those conditions.

Raisins
Tiny fruit battles colon cancer

Raisins are great for snacking. This tiny, dried fruit is full of fiber and antioxidants, as well as tartaric acid. Tartaric acid, found mostly in grapes and their products, works with fiber to make good things happen in your intestines.

Healthy benefits

▶ Gets bowels moving

▶ Prevents colon cancer

▶ Halts hemorrhoids

▶ Protects teeth and gums

Relieves constipation and hemorrhoids. The fiber in raisins softens stool and adds bulk, making waste travel faster through your intestines. This means easier, more regular bowel movements. Reducing the strain of bowel movements can prevent other problems, like hemorrhoids. The researchers found that two servings, or about half a cup, of raisins were all it took to achieve these amazing benefits.

Cuts colon cancer risk. Moving waste through your intestines faster not only relieves constipation, it also fights colon cancer by preventing cancer-causing agents from staying in your intestines too long.

Researchers think fiber and tartaric acid work together to decrease colon cancer risk by diminishing fecal bile acids and some fatty acids, according to a study supported by the California Raisin Marketing Board.

Busts bad bacteria. Earlier studies at Oregon State University also demonstrate raisins' power to kill microbes, like bacteria, viruses, and fungi. The researchers found that ground-up raisins work well as a substitute for sodium nitrite in preserving beef jerky. During digestion, sodium nitrite can break down into cancer-causing chemicals.

Protects teeth and gums. Recent laboratory tests at the University of Illinois in Chicago found that phytochemicals in raisins limit the growth of bacteria that cause dental cavities and gum disease. The researchers say the sugar in raisins is mostly fructose and glucose — not sucrose, which promotes tooth decay.

Almost all of the raisins used in the United States are grown and dried in the sun in California's San Joaquin valley, which also produces about half the world's supply. The best and most-used grape for making raisins is the light green Thompson seedless grape.

3 things you should know about raisins

You can eat raisins by the handful or put them in salads, trail mix, baked goods, hot and cold cereal, or wherever your imagination takes you.

▸ *Keep raisins in an airtight container* in your refrigerator or some other cool area. They also freeze well for long periods of time.

▸ *To plump up raisins for baking,* cover them with hot water for two to five minutes. Use the water in your recipe to save the flavor and the nutrients.

▸ *When chopping raisins,* grease your knife lightly with vegetable oil to keep them from sticking.

Raspberries
Multiple fruit packs antioxidant punch

A raspberry, surprisingly, is not a single fruit, but a cluster. And each tiny little fruit packs a powerful digestive punch. The delicate raspberry is full of cancer-fighting antioxidants and intestinal-cleaning fiber. And its leaves have been used for centuries to treat ailments from constipation to diarrhea.

The individual fruits, called drupelets, connect around a central core, which is why you see it as one berry. But each drupelet has its own seed and skin. Raspberries, especially black ones, look a lot like their cousin the blackberry, but raspberry drupelets are hairy and stick to one another, while blackberries are smooth.

Healthy benefits
▶ Lowers colon cancer risk
▶ Combats constipation
▶ Foils diarrhea
▶ Prevents diverticular disease
▶ Vanquishes nausea
▶ Relieves upset stomach

Wards off colon cancer. Every time you enjoy a raspberry's sweet but subtly tart taste, you may be helping your body fight cancer, according to researchers at Ohio State University. In one study, scientists infected rats with colon cancer and fed some of them black raspberries. The rats developed 80 percent fewer malignant tumors than those kept on a regular diet.

The researchers believe it was antioxidants such as anthocyanins, phenols, and vitamins A, C, E and folic acid in the raspberries that made the difference. They found black raspberries have 11 percent more antioxidants than blueberries and 40 percent more than strawberries. All three berries are among the top 10 foods with the most antioxidants.

Red raspberries are a primary source of the phenolic compound ellagic acid, an important antioxidant whose exact role in cancer prevention is still being studied. One study has shown it can disintegrate cervical cancer cells in a test tube in 48 to 72 hours. Although claims about the effectiveness of ellagic acid supplements are mostly unproven, the polyphenols in raspberries add a lot to the overall antioxidant power of raspberries.

Prevents constipation and diverticulosis. Another raspberry strength is fiber — 8 grams of it in a cup of raw raspberries. Beans and grains have more dietary fiber than these juicy morsels, but the only fruit with more fiber is deglet noor dates. Adding raspberries to your diet will go a long way toward preventing constipation and diverticular disease.

Strikes back at diarrhea and nausea. The fruit of the raspberry isn't the only way this thorny shrub can help you, either. Raspberry leaves are an herbal remedy for diarrhea and other intestinal disorders, including upset stomach, nausea, and vomiting.

Steep two teaspoons of raspberry leaves in boiling water for a soothing tea you can drink up to three times a day — but don't overdo it. Stronger brews may actually provoke nausea and diarrhea in some people. Some herbalists combine raspberry leaves with ginger and dried mint.

Although raspberry tea has long been used to soothe the stomach, little research exists to show why or how well it actually works. Scientists do know the leaves are rich in tannins, which have astringent qualities that are helpful for diarrhea. Their soluble pectin fiber and flavonoids also contribute to good overall intestinal health.

> ## Word to the wise
>
> Fresh raspberries are quite perishable, so use them as soon as possible to ensure the best flavor and nutrient content — and be on the lookout for soft, shriveled, or moldy berries. You can also buy them frozen or in jams, jellies, and juices. Just be aware of added sugar, and remember that processing may destroy some of the vitamin C.

4 things you should know about raspberries

You have to be quick when shopping for fresh raspberries because they don't last long. Here are some tips to help you enjoy them more.

▸ *Shop for fully ripe raspberries* that are aromatic, firm, plump, brightly colored, and have no cores. The core of a ripe raspberry remains attached to the plant, leaving the berry hollow. So, if you find a raspberry with its core intact, that means it was not fully ripe when picked. And raspberries don't ripen after they're picked.

▶ **Handle raspberries gently.** They are very fragile. Wash them quickly in cold water just before using, drain well, and let them air dry, or pat them softly with a paper towel. Don't let them get water soaked or sit at room temperature too long.

▶ **Look for recipes that use raspberry sauce** to top off baked goods and fruit compotes with mouth-watering elegance. Eat them plain, mix them into cereal and yogurt, or use them in salad dressings.

▶ **Freeze raspberries** by placing them in a single layer on a cookie tray. After they're frozen, store them in a sealable plastic bag in the freezer.

Rhubarb
Unusual veggie aids digestion

Rhubarb is a vegetable that thinks it's a fruit, even though its stalks look like red celery. If you accidentally grab a stalk of rhubarb thinking it's celery, you'll realize your mistake as soon as it touches your tongue. Few food plants are as tart as rhubarb. Thankfully, cooking and sweetening can tame the tartness. In fact, it's a popular pie filling.

Healthy benefits

▶ Cures constipation

▶ Does away with diarrhea

▶ Aids digestion

Rhubarb roots have been harvested for centuries because of their medicinal value, but they usually come from varieties grown only in China and Tibet. The stalks of those varieties aren't eaten.

The rhubarb grown and eaten in America and Europe has a powerful taste and potent nutritional punch. A single cup, raw and diced, contains 2 grams of fiber. It's also a good source of vitamin C, magnesium,

Word to the wise

Rhubarb leaves are toxic. They contain dangerous levels of compounds called oxalates. The stalks contain oxalate, too, but in safe amounts. Oxalates can contribute to kidney stone formation, so avoid eating rhubarb if you suffer from kidney disease or urinary problems. If you grow rhubarb, just trim the leaves as you harvest the stalks, then toss them in the compost. They won't hurt garden soil.

vitamin K, calcium, potassium, and manganese. Rhubarb also contains potent phytochemicals called polyphenols and tannins.

Improves digestion. Rhubarb benefits digestion from the moment it enters your mouth. It stimulates your taste buds with its pleasantly bitter flavor, making your mouth feel clean and refreshed. Once it reaches your stomach, rhubarb's digestive benefits really kick in — stimulating the production of gastric juices and improving digestion. It also helps control the absorption of fat in the intestines.

Relieves constipation and diarrhea. The phenol anthraquinone glycosides gives rhubarb stalks their red color and act as a laxative. In fact, they are the same compounds found in other laxative herbs, like cascara and senna. The tannins, on the other hand, help stop diarrhea.

The effects of rhubarb root extract have received lots of attention in scientific literature. Low doses seem to relieve diarrhea, while higher doses help keep you regular. But before you head to the herb shop, consider this — the same phytochemicals contained in the roots are found in smaller amounts in the edible stalks. Plus, you'll get vitamins, minerals, and fiber not found in the extract.

4 things you should know about rhubarb

Not many people are familiar with this unusual vegetable. Here are a few things you should know.

▶ *Go easy on the sweeteners.* Remedy rhubarb's tartness without white sugar. Try alternative sweeteners, like honey or maple syrup. Cooking it calms the tartness a little. Then you can add enough sweetener to suit you.

▶ *Enhance rhubarb's flavor* by stewing it in orange or pineapple juice or with sweet fruits, like apples or strawberries.

▶ *Don't stew rhubarb in aluminum* or cast-iron cookware. Because it's acidic, you could end up with a blackened pot and black rhubarb.

A half-cup of unsweetened, frozen, cooked rhubarb only has 29 calories. The same amount sweetened has 139.

▶ *Preserve rhubarb's natural color.* Parboil it for 30 seconds before you freeze it.

Rice
Remember this grain for regularity

The first people to enjoy rice were probably those living in southern Asia and parts of Africa. But now, thanks to centuries of commerce, it has become popular throughout the world.

Healthy benefits

▶ Conquers constipation

▶ Reduces colon cancer risk

▶ Calms colitis

▶ Tames diarrhea

▶ Evades celiac disease

A look at any food pyramid will give you a snapshot of rice's role in good nutrition. You'll see that whole grains, including brown rice, are an essential part of a healthy diet.

Rice grains comes in three lengths — short, medium, and long. And there are varieties of each — arborio, basmati, jasmine, texmati, and wehani, to name a few. They each have their own flavors, textures, and aromas. And each variety is available in brown and white.

Brown rice is the basic "whole grain" of the rice world. Only its outer husk has been removed, leaving its nutritious bran, germ, and endosperm intact. White rice has those parts removed by additional milling. One result of this processing is that white rice can have up to six times less fiber.

Curbs constipation. Even though white rice loses out in the milling process, it's usually "enriched," or fortified with vitamins and minerals. But enrichment can't replace the bran, the part that makes rice so good for normal digestive health. Bran is the "broom" that sweeps your digestive tract clean of harmful cells. It is also the fiber that helps prevent constipation.

Defends against colon cancer. What's more, rice contains "resistant starch" — starches that withstand stomach acid and reach the bowel undigested. This encourages the growth of beneficial bacteria that keep your bowel healthy. Resistant starch may also help protect you from colon cancer.

Soothes diarrhea and colitis. Both white and whole-grain brown rice provide easily digestible starch for people who have diarrhea or colitis. Yet, white rice is better for treating diarrhea than whole-grain rice. In fact, it's one of the four recommended foods in the BRAT (bananas, rice, applesauce, toast) eating plan to help your body recover from diarrhea. Rice is gentle on your digestive system, wholesome and nutritious, low in fat, and rich in complex carbohydrates, vitamins, and minerals — just what the doctor ordered for people suffering with these conditions.

Sidesteps celiac disease. And rice, both brown and white, provides grain nourishment for people with Celiac disease who can't tolerate gluten, the protein found in most other grains.

Word to the wise

Great-tasting rice mixes are available at any grocery store. But beware! They're loaded with sodium. So why not make your own? You can create savory rice dishes by mixing plain rice with your favorite herbs and spices. Your rice-ipe will taste just as good as any you'll find in a box, and it will be better for you, too.

6 things you should know about rice

You can enjoy rice as a side dish or as a mainstay of meals like stir-fries and paella. Here's how to make the most of this grain.

▸ **Store rice in an airtight container.** Brown rice has a shelf life of about 6 months but will last longer in the refrigerator. White rice will keep up to a year.

▸ **Don't rinse white rice** before cooking, or you'll wash off the added nutrients. To keep it from sticking, avoid stirring during cooking.

▸ **Include leafy green vegetables,** like spinach, in your meals with rice. The amino acids in rice complement those in the greens to form complete proteins.

▸ **Soak brown rice before you cook it** for a nutritional boost. A Japanese study found it makes the grain germinate, giving you higher levels of fiber, nutrients, and phytochemicals.

▸ **Cook rice in a vegetable, beef, or chicken stock** for low-fat, low-calorie flavor.

▸ **Add rice bran to baked goods** and other foods. An ounce contains up to 8 grams of fiber, as well as protein, thiamin, niacin, magnesium, and iron. Use it like wheat germ, and sprinkle it on your cereal, salad, or yogurt.

How did a processed food like white rice end up being cheaper than brown rice, its more nutritious whole-grain twin? Seems like processing would make it cost more. Early on, white rice actually was more expensive. But its longer shelf life, quicker cooking time, and mild flavor made it very popular. As demand rose, prices fell, in spite of the extra processing. Unfortunately, it was later determined that eating white rice as a main staple in the diet causes vitamin-deficiency diseases, such as beriberi and pellagra.

Rosemary
Spicy herb fights harmful intruders

According to an old English myth, rosemary will grow in a garden only if the mistress of the house is really the master. Whether that's true or not, rosemary can certainly help you master your digestive health.

Healthy benefits

▸ Relieves indigestion

▸ Controls gas

▸ Calms intestinal spasms

▸ Thwarts food poisoning

Rosemary is one of the oldest known herbs used for medicine. It originally came from the Mediterranean area, which is why the spice is such a common ingredient in recipes from that region.

Fights cancer. Rosemary has a hefty amount of flavonoids and other powerful antioxidants, like polyphenols, to help it do this. Ninety percent of the antioxidants in rosemary extract are carnosol and carnosic acid. Both are powerful chemicals that scavenge your body for cancer-causing free radicals.

Caffeic acid and rosmarinic acid are two more powerful antioxidants in rosemary extract that help fight cancer. On top of its antioxidant effect, rosemary extract causes your body to make quinone reductase, an enzyme that destroys harmful cancer-causing substances.

But that's not all, of course. Rosemary benefits your digestive tract while it helps protect you from cancer.

Defends against food poisoning. Like many other herbs and spices, rosemary can kill harmful bacteria. Food is more likely to spoil in warm temperatures, so people who lived in hot climates before refrigeration would put a lot of spices, like rosemary, in their food. That's why spicy food is so popular in warm places like South America and southern Europe.

Rosemary oil, in particular, can kill several types of bacteria known for spoiling meat, including *Staphylococcus aureus* and *E. coli.* By getting rid of those tiny invaders, rosemary helps keep you safe from food poisoning.

The spice can also kill certain types of viruses and fungi. Yeast, for example, is on rosemary's hit list. Many herbal experts recommend rosemary oil capsules to treat an overgrowth of yeast in the intestines.

Eases indigestion, gas, and intestinal spasms. Your intestines can benefit from rosemary in another way, too. In medical experiments, rosemary eased spasms in the small intestine. What's more, the German Commission E, well-respected herbal medicine experts and a good resource for the risks and benefits of herbs, has approved rosemary leaf tea for treatment of indigestion, gas, and bloating.

Word to the wise

Rosemary oil can be toxic, especially if you take more than the recommended dose or don't dilute the extract according to the directions on the label. An overdose could irritate your stomach and intestines and damage your kidneys. Many herbal experts suggest playing it safe and taking rosemary oil in the form of enteric-coated capsules. Just follow the directions carefully. To be extra safe, rosemary tea, approved by the German Commission E, may be a better choice.

3 things you should know about rosemary

Working rosemary into your diet can be a tasty way to protect yourself from a variety of health problems. Follow these tips for healthful, not to mention delicious, results.

▸ *Throw some fresh rosemary into your favorite recipes.* It adds a nice flavor to meats, baked goods, and vegetables, like parsnips, peas, potatoes, broccoli, mushrooms, and spinach.

▸ *Use fresh herbs whenever possible.* Herbal experts say fresh herbs are better cancer fighters than the dried variety. It only takes about one teaspoon of rosemary leaf a day to get those health benefits.

▸ *Make rosemary tea* by putting two teaspoons of rosemary leaves in a cup of boiling water. Let it steep for 10 to 15 minutes, then strain. Drink it three times a day.

Salmon
Amazing fish keeps colon in the pink

Salmon is good for you. This popular fish is rich in omega-3 fatty acids. Scientists think they play an important role in brain and visual function, and they help keep your immune system strong.

Healthy benefits
▸ Protects against colon cancer
▸ Calms ulcerative colitis
▸ Prevents flare-ups of Crohn's disease

But did you know that salmon and other seafood is good for your intestines, too? Ongoing research into fish oil shows it may protect you from colon cancer and ease the effects of inflammatory bowel diseases, like Crohn's disease and ulcerative colitis.

Thwarts colon cancer. Researchers have found that fish oil seems to protect against colon cancer, while other oils — those with omega-6 fatty acids — actually promote the disease. They believe the balance of fatty acids in individual cells can determine whether they grow into a tumor or not.

Your body needs both omega-3 fatty acids and omega-6 fatty acids, but it's not good when they get out of balance. When omega-3s break down, their by-products seem to thwart certain kinds of cancer, but some omega-6 by-products might promote cancer.

Unfortunately, your body gets a lot more omega-6 fatty acids because they are found in significant amounts in most vegetable oils, egg yolks, meat, and margarine. And don't eat too many peanuts. They also contain omega-6s. Eating seafood instead of saturated fat raises omega-3s, while lowering omega-6s, giving your body a more even ratio of these essential fatty acids, called "essential" because your body can't make them.

Quiets Crohn's disease. Fish oil also has anti-inflammatory properties that might help people with inflammatory bowel disease. A study of people with Crohn's disease showed that those who took low-dose fish oil capsules for a year had fewer relapses than those who didn't. Fish oil seemed to have this effect because it kept inflammation from flaring up, which may also help sufferers of ulcerative colitis.

Settles down ulcerative colitis. Corticosteroids can effectively control ulcerative colitis inflammation, but doctors worry about their many long-term side effects. A study used fish oil to help people with ulcerative colitis get along with fewer drugs.

Researchers at The Cleveland Clinic found that people with ulcerative colitis who took a supplement containing fish oil, soluble fiber, and antioxidants didn't need as many corticosteroids. In some cases, the supplements kept the disease under control without the side effects of traditional therapies.

Word to the wise

Be careful if you're considering taking cod liver oil supplements instead of eating more salmon. Cod liver oil is naturally rich in vitamins A and D. Vitamin A, and to a lesser extent vitamin D, can be toxic in large doses — although very beneficial at recommended levels (no more than about two or three capsules of cod liver oil a day for adults). Other sources of fish oil do not contain potentially toxic amounts of vitamins A and D. Fish oil is also a natural blood thinner. If you are taking prescription blood-thinning medications, like warfarin, talk with your doctor before trying fish oil supplements.

Fish have become the main food sources of contaminants like mercury and polychlorinated biphenyls (PCBs). The U.S. Food and Drug Administration and the Environmental Protection Agency have published guidelines to help consumers avoid mercury. Here's what their experts say.

▸ Most people can safely eat two 6-ounce servings of salmon a week.

▸ Check local advisories about the safety of fish caught in nearby lakes, rivers, and coastal waters. Otherwise, eat no more than 6 ounces of fish caught from local waters, and eat no other fish that week.

▸ Young children and women who are pregnant, nursing, or may become pregnant should not eat shark, swordfish, king mackerel, or tilefish because they contain high levels of mercury.

Although salmon is very low in mercury, researchers discovered that farmed salmon is higher in PCBs and other toxins than wild salmon. And tests showed that farm-raised Atlantic salmon were the worst offenders. Because PCBs may cause cancer, eating one serving of farmed salmon per month might cause one person out of every 100,000 people to get cancer sometime during his life. That's around 1,000 out of every 100 million people. But that doesn't mean you can't eat salmon again.

Quality salmon doesn't smell fishy. It has a mild aroma similar to fresh fruit. Salmon steaks and fillets should be moist and clear with a deep salmon-pink color. If you buy a whole fish, look for bright, almost lifelike eyes and reddish gills. Fresh salmon flesh is firm and will give slightly when you press it, then spring back into shape.

Oceans Alive, a campaign of the nonprofit Environmental Defense Network, points out that farmed Atlantic salmon are commonly found in grocery stores. But they suggest selecting the low-in-contaminants Alaskan salmon varieties, such as chum, coho, pink, or sockeye. These varieties are safe enough to eat daily.

In fact, the Center for Science and the Public Interest reports that most canned salmon is the wild kind, usually from Alaska, but read the labels to make sure the salmon is one of the wild Alaskan types. And don't forget that out-of-season fresh salmon filets and "Atlantic" salmon may have high levels of contaminants because they are from fish farms.

Your best bet for avoiding toxins may be fish oil supplements. Many are purified to remove contaminants. Consumer Labs, an independent reviewer of consumer products, tested over 40 supplements and found that none of them contained unsafe levels of mercury, PCBs, or even dioxins, another toxin sometimes found in fish.

Environmental Defense surveyed 75 makers of fish oil supplements to gather product quality data. They found that the majority purify their products until the supplement meets rigorous safety standards. Before you try fish oil supplements, talk with your doctor to find out what dosage is right for you, especially if you want to try them for a particular health problem.

3 things you should know about salmon

Salmon cooks quickly, which makes it an easy, no fuss weekday supper or weekend entrée. You can bake, broil, grill, steam, fry, or poach it. No matter how you fix it, here are some tips to make sure your salmon is delicious.

- ▸ *Don't overcook salmon.* It's done when the meat changes color and gets flaky. It keeps cooking after you turn off the heat, so watch closely. Even a minute too long will rob salmon of some of its texture and flavor. Use this rule of thumb — cook salmon about 10 minutes for each inch of thickness.

- ▸ *Leave the skin on* salmon while it cooks. The skin helps hold the fish together, keeps in the flavor and juices, and falls off easily after cooking.

- ▸ *Put your favorite seasonings* in the body cavity and cook the salmon whole, without removing the bone or the skin. When it's done, peel off the skin, eat the top layer of meat, and lift out the skeleton.

Spinach
Battle cancer with a leafy green

Spinach has long ranked near the top of the garden-vegetable charts. Loved for its taste and nutritional value, spinach is also easy to grow — even in mid-winter when only the hardiest of greens will survive.

Healthy benefits

▶ Reduces colon cancer risk

▶ Guards against stomach cancer

Spinach comes in three varieties. The most common is Savoy, known for its crisp, creased, curly leaves, and springy texture. Semi-savoy is similar, just a little less crinkly and creased. Smooth-leaf spinach has flat and unwrinkled leaves, which makes them much easier to wash.

Spinach shares hints of its cousins' flavors — the tartness of beet greens and the saltiness of chard. You might describe spinach as sweet and mild when it's eaten as a salad green, acidic and robust when it's cooked.

Spinach is a great source of antioxidants, such as beta carotene, vitamin C, and vitamin E. It's also rich in folate, an important B vitamin, and lutein, a phytochemical believed to play a role in eye health. This leafy green contains more protein than almost any other vegetable. Although spinach protein lacks one of the essential amino acids, that missing ingredient is available in rice and other grains — which means they're great to serve together.

Battles colon cancer odds. What spinach does for your digestive tract is extraordinary. It protects the cells lining the colon from damage by free radicals, which helps prevent colon cancer. Spinach performs its digestive wonders with an arsenal of antioxidants like vitamin C and beta carotene. Its folate helps prevent DNA damage and dangerous mutations in colon cells — even after those cells have been exposed to cancer-causing chemicals.

Helps prevent stomach cancer. Studies show this green wonder also decreases the risk of stomach cancer. In fact, one Korean study suggested that eating spinach and cabbage reduced the risk of stomach cancer, while eating broiled meats and salty foods increased the risk.

Not everyone should eat spinach in Popeye quantities. It also contains oxalates, acids that in high amounts can contribute to gout, cause trouble if you're anemic, lessen your ability to absorb certain minerals, aggravate gallbladder problems, and play a role in forming kidney stones. But if you eat high-calcium foods when eating foods containing oxalates, the calcium may help bind the oxalates and keep them from being absorbed.

Some experts say you should take calcium supplements within a couple of hours of eating high-oxalate foods. At least one study has suggested that taking calcium supplements may help bind oxalates. One research team has even suggested that the safety or suitability of supplements may be determined by diet and other factors. Since you have so many things to consider, talk with your doctor about what is right for you.

Get more bang for your buck by buying spinach grown during the winter months. Researchers have found that spinach harvested in March has twice the cancer-stopping antioxidant activity of spinach harvested in December. They theorize the tougher, colder conditions may stimulate the production of even more protective phytochemicals.

5 things you should know about spinach

Spinach is available year round, but its best seasons are late fall and spring. That's when it's freshest and has the best flavor.

- ▶ *Wash fresh-picked spinach well.* Dirt loves to lodge in its crinkly leaves. But wait to wash until you're ready to eat it. It will wilt if you store it wet in the refrigerator.

- ▶ *Eat fresh spinach soon.* The longer it sits, the greater its loss of folates and carotenoids — even if it's just a few days.

Refrigeration helps some, but those nutrients will last only about eight days after the leaves have been picked.

- ▶ *Crisp the leaves for salads* by washing them and drying them in a salad spinner. Then wrap in paper towels, stick in a plastic bag, and chill in the refrigerator.

- ▶ *Steam spinach for 5 to 10 minutes* for an easy side dish. It's even better than microwaving because hardly any nutrients are lost.

- ▶ *Add a little olive oil* or other healthy fat to spinach when you cook it. Your body will have an easier time absorbing its carotenoids — beta carotene, lutein, and zeaxanthin. In fact, cooking makes all this vegetable's antioxidants easier to absorb.

Tea
Surprising benefits of tea

Tea is still a popular beverage after thousands of years, and it's no wonder when you consider all its benefits.

The Chinese are credited with discovering this delicious drink in 2737 B.C. by a fortunate accident. Emperor Shen-Nung was boiling water on his terrace when leaves from a nearby bush blew over and fell into the water. He tried it and thought it tasted great. Before long, people all over China and the rest of East Asia were making tea.

Healthy benefits

- ▶ Quiets gastritis
- ▶ Protects against stomach cancer
- ▶ Staves off esophageal cancer
- ▶ Resists colon cancer
- ▶ Averts rectal cancer

According to Indian legend, Siddhartha Gautama Buddha was the first to bring tea to India after his travels through China. The Dutch and British started importing tea during the 17th century, but they preferred black tea, unlike the green variety more common in the East. Even now, black tea is more popular than green tea in Western nations.

The leaves of green and black tea come from the same plant, *Camellia sinensis*. The difference is in how they're prepared. Green tea leaves are steamed right after they've been picked, which helps preserve the antioxidants. For black tea, the leaves are allowed to ferment a while.

A third kind of tea, Red Bush tea, is gaining popularity. Known in its native South Africa as "Rooibos" (ROY-boss), which is Dutch for "red bush," Red Bush tea comes from the plant *Aspalathus linearis*, a shrub with needle-like leaves. Living up to its name, Red Bush tea has a reddish-brown color and a strong taste. It has the antioxidants of black tea and more, but none of the caffeine. Red Bush tea is also low in oxalic acid, which can be harmful to your kidneys.

Word to the wise

Green tea does not have as much caffeine as coffee or even black tea, but it still has some. If caffeine irritates your stomach, switch to decaffeinated black or green tea, so you can get all the antioxidants without the unpleasant side effects. Or just drink Red Bush tea, which has no caffeine at all.

Black, green, and Red Bush teas are all rich in polyphenols called catechins, which are antioxidants. Green tea has the most catechins of the three. That's because soon after tea leaves are harvested, an enzyme called polyphenol oxidase changes the catechins into another chemical. This chemical change is what causes the color of the leaves to turn from green to dark brown. Green tea, on the other hand, is steamed right away, which stops the enzyme before it can change anything.

Cools gastritis. You may never have thought of drinking tea to soothe your stomach, but that's one of its surprising benefits. If acid gives your stomach grief, try sipping green tea instead of soda. Drinking tea regularly helps ease painful gastritis, or inflammation of the stomach lining, while soda only makes it worse.

In fact, a University of California study of 600 Chinese men and women revealed people who frequently drank green tea were half as likely to suffer from gastritis. Perhaps that's because the antioxidants in tea can help prevent not only gastritis, but also the cancer-causing lesions that come with it.

Shields against stomach cancer. The University of California study made another discovery, too. It found that frequent green tea drinkers were half as likely to get stomach cancer, the second most common cancer in the world. But there's even more. In a 12-year study, a group of researchers kept tabs on some men who regularly drank tea. The researchers found these tea fans also had half the chance of getting stomach cancer as men who didn't drink tea.

The Japanese have been perfecting the art of tea drinking for centuries. Getting together with friends for tea can be a casual thing or a formal event, called a "chaji." This ceremony can last from three to five hours and may include a meal with several courses and a break to relax in a garden.

Deters colon, rectal, and esophageal cancers. Tea may help prevent more than just stomach cancer. Another study showed drinking as little as one cup of tea a week may cut your chances of getting cancer of the esophagus in half. Still more studies have shown that black tea may be effective at fighting colon and rectal cancer.

So take the time to relax often with a cup of your favorite tea. You'll be doing your body a favor.

5 things you should know about tea

Make the most of your tea-drinking experience by following these helpful tips.

▶ *Look for Red Bush and green tea in grocery stores* and health food stores. Red Bush tea from South Africa may be more potent than the varieties grown in other African countries. You can get it loose or in tea bags. If you buy it loose, look for leaves with an even color and delicate, rather than strong, aroma. You can find black tea easily in a supermarket.

▶ *Steep green tea and black tea for about three minutes* in water that's hot but not boiling. Boiling water destroys some of the antioxidants in tea. Red Bush tea is slightly different. The longer you steep it, especially in very hot water, the more antioxidants you get. Anywhere from five to 10 minutes should do the trick.

▶ *Drink green tea before it cools* and turns a darker brown. The changing color is a sign the antioxidants no longer work.

▶ *Try supplements* if you don't care for the taste of green tea. These capsules contain extracts of the polyphenols you usually find in green tea. Some capsules can give you as many polyphenols as four cups of green tea.

▶ *Drink Brassica teas with added antioxidants* for extra healing punch. Black, green, and Red Bush teas from Brassica Protection Products have Sulforaphane Glucosinolate (SGS) added to them. SGS is an antioxidant found in broccoli that helps prevent cancer and may help kill bacteria that cause gastritis or other serious digestive problems. For more information about Brassica teas, call toll-free at 877-747-1277 or visit *www.brassica.com* on the Internet.

Tomatoes
Summer favorite gets tough on disease

The tomato is one of those foods it's hard not to like. You can eat it fresh from the garden in the summer, or use it throughout the year in salads, sandwiches, soups, and stews. Tomato sauce is an essential ingredient in all types of foods, and ketchup can top everything from burgers to eggs.

Healthy benefits

▶ Protects against digestive cancers

▶ Prevents duodenal ulcers

Whatever way you enjoy tomatoes, you reap their healthy benefits. They are rich in lycopene and other antioxidants that help protect you from stomach, colorectal, and esophageal cancer as well as heart disease, prostate cancer, and osteoporosis.

Italian cuisine is famous for using tomatoes, but they started out in western South America, not Italy. The Mexicans learned to cultivate them, and Spanish conquistadors took them to Europe. Tomatoes spread through Europe, appeared in Italy during the 16th century, and then came to North America with the colonists who settled in Virginia.

But tomatoes were grown more as an ornamental plant than for food. Europeans considered the fruit poisonous since the plant is a member of the deadly nightshade family. It was not until the late 1800s, after selective breeding had removed most solanine, a natural toxin, from tomatoes, that people actually began to enjoy eating them.

Today, tomatoes of many varieties, shapes, sizes, and colors are grown and eaten all over the world. It's a garden favorite sold fresh, canned, and in products like ketchup and tomato sauce.

Cuts the risk of cancer. The tomato's high level of lycopene is one reason researchers believe people who eat a lot of tomatoes and tomato products have less cancer. Among gastrointestinal ailments, researchers have found the strongest benefit for stomach cancer. Tomatoes also may decrease the risk of cancer in the colon, rectum, and esophagus.

But lycopene may not be the only reason for tomatoes' anti-cancer qualities. Scientists recognize that cancer defense may come from other antioxidants working together with lycopene. Other studies show the protection increases even more when tomatoes are eaten with garlic.

Puts a stop to ulcers. Even without lycopene, tomatoes would be a great choice. They are rich in vitamin C, fiber, and beta carotene, the plant substance your body turns into vitamin A. Recent research has found that fiber from fruits and vegetables, along with vitamin A, reduces the risk of duodenal ulcers. These are bleeding sores that develop in the upper part of your small intestine.

Your body absorbs more lycopene and other antioxidants from cooked tomatoes, especially if a small amount of olive or canola oil is used in the process. That's why you get more out of tomato sauce and tomato paste than from tomatoes fresh off the vine.

6 things you should know about tomatoes

Regular fruits have dessert-quality sweetness, but tomatoes act more like vegetables. Cooking brings out their sweetness and tempers their acidity. Here are some tips to get the most out of tomatoes.

▸ **Shop for tomatoes that are firm,** heavy, and smell like a tomato. Unripe tomatoes have no odor. You'll find the best tomato flavor in mid to late summer.

▸ **Don't buy tomatoes from the refrigerator case.** Temperatures below 55 degrees stop the ripening process and kill the taste and texture of tomatoes. Don't put tomatoes in your refrigerator at home, either, unless they're so ripe they'll spoil if you don't.

▸ **Ripen your tomatoes at room temperature,** but not on your sunny windowsill. To speed up ripening, put them in a paper bag with a banana, which gives off a gas that speeds up the process.

▸ **Use cooked tomatoes for the most health benefits.** Surprisingly, cooked tomato products like ketchup and tomato sauce offer even more protection than raw tomatoes. Processing and cooking helps break down cell walls in the tomato, making it easier for your body to absorb the nutrients.

▸ **Avoid aluminum pots and pans** when cooking tomatoes. The reaction between tomatoes' acid and aluminum produces a bad taste that could also lead to consuming harmful amounts of aluminum.

▸ **Eat the tomato itself** rather than take supplements containing the same nutrients to reap the most benefit.

Turmeric
Tame troubling tummy problems

Spicing up your life could actually end indigestion, nausea, and bloating, among other ills. Turmeric comes from the plant *Curcuma longa,* a member of the ginger family native to India and China. People harvest the plant's rhizome, then clean, boil, and dry it to make turmeric spice.

Healthy benefits

▸ Cools heartburn

▸ Ends indigestion

▸ Nixes nausea

▸ Eliminates gas

▸ Curbs colon cancer

▸ Stymies stomach cancer

▸ Fends off IBD

You probably know it from eating out. Turmeric is a main ingredient in curry, a blend of spices used heavily in Indian and Asian food. But it does more than add flavor, and that may be what makes it so popular.

Banishes heartburn, gas, and indigestion. Turmeric helps relieve symptoms of heartburn, nausea, and bloating that follows a fatty meal. These symptoms, along with light-colored stools, could indicate poor bile flow from your liver to gallbladder. Bile is an important digestive juice. Too little of it, and you'll feel dyspeptic — bloated and sick to your stomach — after normal-size meals.

Turmeric contains bitter compounds that stimulate digestive juices, including bile. Bitters prompt the liver to pump out more bile, which helps you digest food better without uncomfortable indigestion, gas, and other intestinal problems. In fact, some evidence shows curcumin, one of the main compounds in turmeric, nearly doubles the amount of bile the liver puts out. Plus, turmeric is a natural antacid and anti-flatulent.

Curbs colon cancer risk. Curcumin could erase stomach and colon cancer, too. This compound gives turmeric its bright yellow color, and it is an antioxidant powerhouse. In lab studies, curcumin suppressed the growth of cancer cells and easily destroyed them.

So far, scientists have only tested turmeric's cancer-fighting abilities in animals and test tubes. Human studies are in the works. In the meantime, experts say if you like the spice, go ahead and enjoy it. You just might ward off cancer in the process.

Helps calm IBD. New lab studies also found curcumin protected the colons of mice and prevented inflammatory bowel disease (IBD) symptoms, such as diarrhea, after scientists tried to give the animals colitis. These researchers believe curcumin's combination of antioxidant and anti-inflammatory powers may put a lid on the oxidative stress, inflammation, and out-of-control immune response that characterize IBD.

You can get turmeric just by eating food made with curry. Look for curry dishes in Asian and Indian restaurants, or buy turmeric at your local grocery and add a dash to your own cooking.

Word to the wise

It's paradoxical that something that may help improve the flow of necessary bile from your gallbladder to your small intestine, and possibly help prevent the formation of gallstones, could also aggravate existing gallbladder problems. Even in small amounts, the spice can stir up and aggravate gallstones or blockages in the bile duct, so avoid it if you have these conditions. Stay away from it, as well, if you take a blood-thinning drug, such as Coumadin, warfarin, or NSAIDs, or if you have bleeding problems. The curcumin in turmeric adds to the effect of these medicines.

5 things you should know about turmeric

This spice holds promise for defeating some of your most common stomach ills, but seek out an expert if your symptoms are severe. They could be signs of a more serious condition.

Make your own salt-free curry blend by mixing:

▶ 2 tablespoons each turmeric and ground coriander

▶ 1 tablespoon ground cumin

▶ 2 teaspoons each ground cardamom, ground ginger, and black pepper

▶ 1 teaspoon each powdered cloves, cinnamon, and ground nutmeg

Add a dash of it to seafood, poultry, beef, potato soups, salads, and milk-based cream sauces.

▶ *Make a milk drink* by dissolving 1/4 to 5/8 teaspoon of turmeric in a glass of warm milk, then drink it after or between meals. Don't try to brew a tea with it, though. The spice does not dissolve in water.

▶ *Shop for powdered turmeric* in the spice aisle of the nearest grocery store. Indian grocers and natural food stores may carry fresher spices because they have a faster turnaround.

▶ *Add a dash of black pepper* to turmeric if trying it in food. Piperine, the main phytonutrient in pepper, raises your body's intake of curcumin a whopping 2,000 percent.

▶ *Cook a few dishes* with yellow rice since it contains turmeric.

▶ *Look for turmeric supplements* standardized to contain 400 to 600 milligrams (mg) of curcumin. Experts generally recommend three capsules each day, or between 0.5 grams and 3 grams daily.

Wheat bran
'Bran-tastic' way to battle cancer

Sometimes you don't have to remove the wrapping to get at your present. That's certainly the case with wheat bran, the outer husk of

Healthy benefits

▶ Eliminates constipation

▶ Protects against colon cancer

▶ Helps prevent weight gain

the wheat kernel. Wheat bran is a true gift to your digestive system.

Conquers constipation. Not surprisingly, it's loaded with fiber — a whopping 25 grams per cup, which means good news for your gut. Insoluble fiber, the kind in wheat bran, adds bulk to your stool and dilutes cancer-causing substances that might be in it. It also speeds your stool through the gastrointestinal tract so it's not hanging around causing trouble. This also makes wheat bran good for curing constipation and maintaining a healthy gut.

Blasts tumors. But fiber is not wheat bran's only hero. Wheat bran also has a lot of phytic acid, a substance with antioxidant powers that may stop tumors. Those who doubt fiber's anti-cancer powers point to phytic acid as a possible explanation for wheat bran's effectiveness against colon tumors.

Word to the wise

Wheat bran is not for everyone. Wheat contains gluten, a sticky protein that's dangerous for people with celiac disease or a gluten allergy. If you have a gluten allergy, wheat products could give you cramps, diarrhea, and other problems. Celiac disease is even more serious, and eating wheat could severely damage the lining of your intestines.

If you suffer from irritable bowel syndrome, bran may actually make your symptoms worse. Instead, get your fiber from fresh fruits and vegetables, such as figs, apricots, cantaloupe, and peaches.

Whether it's the fiber or the phytic acid, wheat bran works even better than other cereals. Studies have shown wheat bran can inhibit both colon and other intestinal tumors better than other brans, such as oat or barley.

Helps you stay slim and trim. As an added bonus, bran helps you lose weight — or at least not gain weight. A recent eight-year study found that men who ate the most bran gained 15 percent less weight than those who ate the least. For every 20-gram-per-day increase in bran intake, weight gain decreased by about a pound.

3 things you should know about wheat bran

Wheat bran isn't just for health nuts. Make it a part of your everyday diet — and enjoy a "bran" new, healthier you.

▶ *Find ways to work wheat bran* into your diet. Start your day with a wheat bran cereal. Add unprocessed wheat bran, or miller's bran, to baked goods, like muffins or breads. You can also sprinkle it on cereal or fruit.

▶ *Proceed with caution.* As with any high-fiber food, add wheat bran to your diet gradually. Too much fiber too quickly can cause gas, cramps, bloating, and diarrhea.

▶ *Boost your protection* from colon cancer by teaming wheat bran with other resistant starches, or prebiotics. This type of dietary starch passes undigested through your stomach and small intestine, then settles in your colon, where bacteria tackle it. That produces butyric acid, a fatty acid that helps prevent colon cancer. Good sources of resistant starch and soluble fiber include black beans, kidney beans, peas, lentils, and unprocessed cereal grains, like corn, sorghum, and barley. For more information about prebiotics, see "Another way to keep your gut healthy" in the *Probiotics* section in Chapter 4.

Yogurt
Surprising way to beat gut diseases

Bacteria are more than just bad bugs lurking on doorknobs waiting to make you sick. Some fight on the side of good. Right now, billions of bacteria are living in your intestines helping digest food and protecting you from harmful germs.

Healthy benefits

▶ Battles IBD

▶ Fends off food poisoning

▶ Ditches diarrhea

▶ Prevents colon cancer

▶ Stops stomach ulcers

▶ Eases lactose intolerance

Unfortunately, a round of antibiotics or a poor diet can kill off the good bugs. Without them, bad bacteria invade and take over, triggering all sorts of digestive problems.

Eating yogurt restores your system's natural balance by keeping unfriendly bacteria at bay. The beneficial bacteria in your gut are some of the same kinds used to make yogurt. This treat replenishes the good bugs in your intestines with bacteria that have natural antibiotic and anti-inflammatory powers. Once in your gut, they fight off the troublemakers.

In this case, more is better. The more good bacteria the yogurt contains, the greater chance many will survive the stomach's acid and make it to your intestines. Each milliliter of brand-name yogurt contains around 125 million *L. bulgaricus* bacteria, as well as 125 million *Streptococcus thermophilus* bacteria, two of the friendly species responsible for digestive health. Yogurt manufacturers may also add other kinds of bacteria naturally found in your gut to further boost its healing powers. Thanks to these disease-battling bugs, yogurt may prevent and treat many digestive illnesses.

Word to the wise

Buy yogurt with the "Live and Active Cultures" seal on the carton or the words "active," "live," or "viable" cultures on its label. These phrases promise the product contains living bacteria, the only kind that benefits your digestive system.

For the manufacturer to use these words, the yogurt must contain at least 100 million live bacteria when made, and they must remain alive until its expiration date.

Eases intestinal inflammation. Take the case of *acidophilus*, a bacterium that normally lives in your colon. A round of antibiotics can kill it off, triggering intestinal inflammation accompanied by excessive gas, morning diarrhea, even hemorrhoid pain. Luckily, all of these symptoms respond to yogurt made with active *acidophilus* cultures.

Battles IBD. Fight inflammatory bowel disease (IBD) with this yummy snack. Studies suggest a lack of microflora, the good bacteria in your

Yogurt may have been a mistake. Rumor has it a Turkish nomad first discovered it when the milk in his goatskin bag curdled on a long desert journey.

gut, plays a major role in the development of IBD, including Crohn's disease and ulcerative colitis.

Colon biopsies of people with Crohn's show they have fewer *Lactobacillus* and *Bifidobacterium* microflora than healthy people. Experts think this shortage leaves your digestive lining vulnerable to attack from disease- and inflammation-causing organisms. Yogurt, it seems, may prevent the onset of Crohn's and colitis, as well as ease IBD symptoms.

Fights food poisoning. The live cultures in yogurt may treat, even prevent, this serious illness. This creamy dessert kills bacteria like *Salmonella* and *E. coli* in your colon, common culprits behind food poisoning.

In lab experiments, *Lactobacillus (L.) acidophilus* stopped dangerous strains of *E. coli* and *Salmonella* from gaining a foothold in living cells. In another study, researchers in the Netherlands fed rats either yogurt, milk, or acidified milk. The yogurt-fed rats fought off *Salmonella* infections better than the others. Other lab tests found yogurt killed 11 strains of *Campylobacter jejuni*, another bacterial cause of intestinal problems, in less than 25 minutes.

Puts an end to ulcers. The good bacteria in yogurt also seem to help protect your stomach lining from *H. pylori* bacterium, the kind that causes ulcers and leads to gastritis. Certain yogurt bacteria, such as *L. acidophilus* and *L. gasseri*, actively fight back against *H. pylori* infections. Others destroy bad bacteria linked to gastritis. Yogurt may even ease the side effects of antibiotics used to treat ulcers.

Beats diarrhea. Eat it to treat diarrhea caused by antibiotics or viruses. Experts suggest eating one or two 8-ounce containers of yogurt each day in addition to seeing your doctor.

Goes easy on lactose intolerance. Plus, it's a great source of calcium if you are lactose-intolerant. People lacking the lactase enzyme can often digest yogurt easier than other dairy products. Scientists suspect the active bacterial cultures help your body break down the lactose.

There's more. Epidemiologic studies suggest fermented dairy products could lower your risk of colon cancer. And a new Italian study found that elderly people who ate yogurt had less-severe stomach and intestinal infections and recovered faster than those who didn't.

It's hard to find a better all-around digestive remedy, especially one with no significant side effects. So bone up on the best-tasting tummy tamer money can buy.

5 things you should know about yogurt

It's hard to go wrong with a food that tastes so good and is so good for you. Follow this advice for the most healthful benefits.

▸ *Buy yogurt with the latest expiration date.* The good bacteria weaken as the product ages.

▸ *Store it in the refrigerator* in its original container for up to 10 days.

▸ *Shop for yogurt without added sugar* if you have irritable bowel syndrome (IBS). Many IBS sufferers have trouble absorbing sugar.

▸ *Enjoy it straight from the carton,* add fruit, or mix it with cereal. You can cook with it, too, but heat will kill the helpful bacteria.

▸ *Try frozen yogurt* if you don't like the regular kind, but realize it may have fewer live bacteria and possibly fewer health benefits.

CHAPTER 6

OUT OF EVERY 5,000 PROMISING CHEMICAL COMPOUNDS TESTED, 4,999 don't turn out to be safe and effective enough to become an approved treatment. Similarly, each remedy in this chapter has something controversial about it. For example, some aren't proven to be effective or

Products and therapies: What you should know

won't work for everyone, while others can cause serious side effects. Read on to learn the good, the bad, and the ugly about these products and therapies.

Antacids
Quick way to cool the fire

Antacids used to be simple — two or three brands on the grocery shelf. Pop one and you'd be pain free. Now you have a lot more choices, and that's a good thing. Antacids treat a wide range of digestive troubles. Your doctor may recommend them for:

▸ indigestion

▸ heartburn

▸ gastroesophageal reflux disease (GERD)

▸ ulcers

▸ gastritis

▸ certain kinds of diarrhea and constipation

Some antacids are not safe long-term when taken frequently, and some work better than others, especially for bad cases of acid reflux. Traditional antacids work by neutralizing acid in the esophagus and stomach. Newer antacids, called acid reducers, work by reducing the amount of acid your stomach produces.

The trick is figuring out which tablet, pill, or liquid is best for your heartburn. Basically, you can choose from three kinds.

▸ Traditional acid neutralizers, like Tums, Rolaids, and Maalox

Newer products that reduce stomach acid production include:

▸ Histamine (H_2) blockers, including Pepcid, Zantac, and Tagamet

▸ Proton pump inhibitors (PPIs), such as Prilosec, Prevacid, and Nexium

Traditional antacids, such as Tums, actually neutralize the acid in your stomach, up to 99 percent of it. They raise the pH level in your stomach from around 2, or very acidic, to 3 or 4, which is mildly acidic. A pH of 4 is only 1/100 as acidic as a pH of 2. The upside — they work fast. The downside — they only last a few hours. You can count on them to contain one or more of these ingredients.

▶ **Aluminum and magnesium salts.** These two work well together at calming stomach acid, so products often contain both. Magnesium salts dissolve quickly for fast-acting relief, while aluminum salts break down slowly, for longer-lasting results. Magnesium salts can cause diarrhea, while aluminum salts may triggers constipation. Together, they balance each other out.

▶ **Calcium carbonate.** The active ingredient in Tums and other products, which is basically chalk, has lots going for it — it works fast, is relatively long-lasting, and provides a good, cheap source of calcium. That's important, considering as many as 85 percent of people don't get enough calcium in their diet. And

Avoid milk of magnesia overdose

Is "gastrointestinal hurry" depleting your body of essential nutrients and leaving you feeling tired and worn out? Your body needs magnesium, and magnesium in foods and small amounts of magnesium from supplements may be beneficial. Some over-the-counter antacids contain magnesium, as do certain laxatives and even pain relievers. Take large doses often, and the mineral may build up in your body causing diarrhea. Food rushes through the colon before your gut absorbs all the nutrients, leading to nutritional deficiencies.

Don't poison yourself. Stick with antacid products like Tums, which is entirely calcium carbonate, or Rolaids and Mylanta Supreme, which contain mostly calcium carbonate with relatively small amounts of magnesium. Avoid taking milk of magnesia or products like Maalox and Mylanta Classic, which contain relatively large amounts of magnesium, for more than a week. And never take more than the recommended dose of any antacid.

Traditional antacid tablets work better than liquid antacids, even within the same brand. Oklahoma researchers studied 65 heartburn sufferers and discovered antacid tablets gave greater, longer-lasting relief than the liquids. In fact, the only people with heartburn two hours later were those who used liquid.

Experts suspect the crunched-up tablets stick better to your esophagus, lowering acid levels. Also, chewing them may stimulate the natural antacids in saliva.

antacids that contain mainly calcium carbonate are self-regulating because calcium carbonate only dissolves in an acidic environment. It never completely shuts off the acid in your stomach that is important for digestion and helping to kill harmful bacteria that may be present in food.

Some antacids add the ingredient simethicone, which relieves the uncomfortable symptoms of gas. Maalox and Mylanta Classic (regular and maximum strength) can get rid of diarrhea, intestinal gas, and other disagreeable bowel symptoms, while also lessening your heartburn. Rolaids and the Mylanta Supreme formula, on the other hand, do not contain potentially harmful aluminum salts that, with prolonged use, may deplete calcium and phosphorus from bones and weaken them. Instead, these products contains a small amount of magnesium hydroxide (milk of magnesia) to help balance the possible constipating effect of the main ingredient, calcium carbonate.

Newer acid-reducing drugs are a different kind altogether. Technically, H_2-blockers and PPIs are not antacids. They don't neutralize acid. They lower the amount of acid your stomach produces. This makes them much more powerful than traditional heartburn medicines.

▶ *Histamine blockers* work best for mild to moderate reflux. They block the histamine-2 receptors on the stomach cells that make acid and stop them from producing more. The medicine must get into your bloodstream before it begins to work. So you won't feel relief as quickly as with a regular antacid, but it will last much longer. In fact, you only need one dose twice a day.

Relief from your kitchen cabinet

Sodium bicarbonate is a quick cure for stomach acid, and it costs just pennies. Also known as bicarbonate of soda or baking soda, it acts very fast, producing carbon dioxide gas as a byproduct. You know it's working when you start burping. Warning! Baking powder is different and harmful to take!

Unfortunately, baking soda is also loaded with sodium, which can cause problems for people with high blood pressure or heart failure. Overusing it can also throw off your body's acid-base balance, an extremely serious medical condition. For these reasons, most experts recommend calcium-based antacids, H2 blockers, or PPIs instead.

If you decide to use baking soda, be sure you use it correctly. Take it an hour or two after meals for use as an antacid, not when your stomach is full. You can take a dose every two hours if indigestion persists. But never take more than seven half-teaspoons in a 24-hour period, or three half-teaspoons if you're over 60.

▸ **Proton pump inhibitors (PPIs)** also slash stomach acid. But instead of stopping the cells that make it, they block the cells that pump the acid into your stomach. PPIs are even more powerful than H_2 blockers — one dose is good for the whole day. Doctors often prescribe them for more severe cases of reflux.

Aside from treating heartburn and GERD, experts use H_2 blockers and PPIs to help heal peptic ulcers and esophagitis, or inflammation of the esophagus.

These medicines give ulcers a chance to heal by cutting down the amount of acid your stomach makes for a longer time than regular antacids. Doctors now prescribe a regimen of antibiotics plus a PPI or H_2 to cure ulcers for good.

Sounds great, but this new generation of antacids does have a drawback. Researchers have linked H_2 blockers and PPIs to increased risk for pneumonia, especially in older adults. Apparently, lower levels of acid in the stomach aren't as effective in killing harmful bacteria that may be aspirated from gastric reflux. The risk is small, but tell your doctor if you begin having breathing problems while taking one of these drugs.

And if you haven't talked with your doctor about painful, recurring heartburn — do it now. Antacids may help manage the pain, but they generally don't treat the cause of it. Long-term heartburn does not always indicate a dangerous disease, but antacids can mask serious illnesses. Don't ignore your body's warning signs. See a doctor about chronic heartburn. She can treat it effectively and bring you lasting relief.

6 things you should know about antacids

Antacid tablets are used by millions of people. They couldn't possibly be harmful, right? Medical evidence says that's wrong. The hidden side effects can be dangerous.

Antacids generally are safe if you take them occasionally in small doses, but regular use of large amounts can have dangerous results. Don't poison yourself with over-the-counter antacids. Find out which ones to watch out for.

▶ *If you tend to be constipated,* stick with antacids like Rolaids or Mylanta Supreme that contain some magnesium, but not excessive amounts. If you tend to get diarrhea, choose antacids that are entirely calcium carbonate, like Tums.

▶ *Aluminum hydroxide interferes* with the way your body absorbs calcium, thus weakening your bones. Scientists have begun questioning the safety of aluminum-containing antacids, so avoid using them long-term. Ask your doctor if you are at risk for osteoporosis, and consider a different antacid.

▶ *You can overdose on calcium* just by taking too many antacids. Limit your use to no more than 1,200 milligrams of calcium carbonate, about two Tums, each day.

▶ *Sodium bicarbonate and seltzer-type antacids* are high in sodium, so skip them if you're on a low-sodium diet or have high blood pressure.

▶ *Don't take the maximum dose* of any over-the-counter histamine blocker, like Pepcid or Zantac, for more than two weeks without your doctor's approval.

▶ *All antacids can interact with medications,* some seriously. Remember to tell your doctor if you are taking any medication, and how often.

Aspirin
2-cent solution conquers cancer

Relieve headaches, prevent heart disease, and defend against cancer for just pennies a day. Aspirin and other pain relievers could be the 2-cent colon cleansers that help prevent these cancers.

▶ colon

▶ stomach

▶ throat

▶ mouth

▶ esophageal

Doctors have known for thousands of years about the healing powers of aspirin. Hippocrates first wrote about treating pain and fevers with willow bark, the natural form of aspirin, in the fifth century B.C.

In the 1800s, chemists made salicylic acid from salicin, the active ingredient in willow bark, and used it in high doses to relieve pain and fever. Unfortunately, the acid was tough on tummies, and many people couldn't "stomach" it.

Doctors treated pain, swelling, and fever with willow bark or its extract, aspirin, for more than 2,000 years without knowing how or why it worked. In the early 1970s, British scientist Dr. John Vane and a team of researchers finally solved the mystery of how aspirin worked on cyclooxygenase receptors. They received the Nobel Prize in Medicine in 1982 for their discovery, and Vane was made a British knight.

German chemist Felix Hoffmann remedied the situation in the late 19th century. His father suffered from arthritis but could not handle salicylic acid. Hoffman set out to develop a gentler form of the medicine, one his father could tolerate. He succeeded, and his employer, Friedrich Bayer & Co., dubbed the new drug aspirin and made it famous.

Aspirin, ibuprofen, and naproxen, among others, belong to a class of drugs known as nonsteroidal anti-inflammatory drugs (NSAIDs). These drugs keep an enzyme in your body called cyclooxygenase (COX) from making chemicals known as prostaglandins.

Prostaglandins are messenger molecules that help your body's immune system make repairs and regulate other vital functions. Prostaglandins are neither good nor bad. Your body needs various prostaglandins in proper balance for optimal health.

All prostaglandins are not the same. Some protect the lining of your stomach. Without them, stomach acid erodes the lining, leading to bleeding and ulcers. Other prostaglandins, when produced in excessive amounts, may trigger pain and swelling and seem to stimulate the growth of cancer cells.

COX comes in two forms — COX-1 and COX-2. We need both kinds, but in our modern society, COX-1 makes the generally protective prostaglandins in the stomach, while COX-2 seems to make other prostaglandins throughout the body that may sometimes produce excessive inflammation.

Food provides your body with arachidonic acid, an essential fatty acid. It attaches to COX enzymes, which then use it to make prostaglandins. Aspirin and other NSAIDs plug the hole on COX where arachidonic acid usually attaches, blocking it so COX can't make prostaglandins. Eventually the drugs wear off, your body goes back to making prostaglandins, and you may have to take another dose.

Scientists think putting a damper on prostaglandin production may keep cancerous tumors from forming in the first place.

> ▶ Scientists recently found that taking a daily, low-dose aspirin, 81 milligrams (mg), cut colon cancer risk 19 percent, and this smaller dose was more effective than the regular 325-mg dose. In another study of 90,000 women, researchers discovered that those who took four to six aspirin a week for 20 years lowered their risk of colon cancer 44 percent.

> ▶ Aspirin may prevent other cancers, too. Italian researchers found that, out of 2,700 people, those taking low-dose aspirin regularly for over five years cut their risk of cancer of the esophagus (esophageal cancer) between 20 and 34 percent. Regular, long-term aspirin use also lowered the risk of mouth cancer and throat cancer.

> ▶ Stomach cancer could be next. Chinese scientists analyzed nine studies and found a similar protective effect. These researchers

Word to the wise

Ulcers not caused by *H. pylori* bacteria often erupt from regular use of aspirin and other NSAIDs. NSAIDs block both good and bad effects of prostaglandins. The bad effects can stimulate pain, inflammation, and the growth of cancerous cells. The good effects protect your stomach lining. Taking too much aspirin leaves your stomach and intestinal lining open to injury from stomach acid, which can lead to ulcers and bleeding. However, the danger of taking an 81-mg "baby" aspirin daily is small.

think how long you take NSAIDs may be more important than the size of the dose. This is good news because large doses of NSAIDs are associated with greater risk of stomach bleeding.

Experts don't know yet how long you have to take aspirin to reap a protective benefit, but one thing is certain — talk with your doctor before deciding to take aspirin or other NSAIDs to prevent any form of cancer. These drugs can have serious side effects, especially with long-term use.

A newer class of drugs called COX-2 inhibitors (Vioxx, Celebrex) only block the COX-2 enzyme. They were advertised by the drug companies that developed them as superior to aspirin and other NSAIDs that block both the COX-1 and COX-2 enzymes.

But the scientists who created COX-2 drugs didn't know as much about the immune system as they thought they did. Taking COX-2 drugs has now been associated with a large increase in heart attacks among users, leading to the withdrawal of one of these drugs, Vioxx, from the market.

Because they block COX-1 enzymes that produce prostaglandins, which protect the stomach, NSAIDs such as aspirin can thin the protective lining in your stomach, allowing stomach acid to damage the lining and leading to ulcers and bleeding. Small doses of aspirin, such as 81-mg low-dose aspirin, are safe for most people, but anyone with a history of stomach bleeding or ulcers should avoid any form of aspirin and most other NSAIDs.

8 things you should know about aspirin — and other NSAIDs

Aspirin has the best long-term record of all NSAIDs for greatest benefits with generally lowest side effects. But ibuprofen and naproxen may be better for some people. Save your stomach from the wear and tear of long-term NSAID use with a few helpful hints.

▶ *Make NSAIDs easier* on your stomach by taking them with food.

▸ **Chew an antacid** after taking aspirin to settle stomach upset.

▸ **Try vitamin C.** Evidence suggests taking vitamin C with aspirin may protect your stomach.

▸ **Check the expiration date** and toss aspirin if they're past their prime. Aspirin slowly reverts to salicylic acid over time, which is much tougher on your stomach.

▸ **Talk with your doctor** before using aspirin, especially if you are taking blood-thinning medications or antidepressant drugs. Both increase your risk of stomach bleeding when combined with NSAIDs.

▸ **Avoid taking aspirin if you have a sensitive stomach or ulcers.** Taking even one baby aspirin daily can cause ulcers if you are at high risk for stomach problems.

▸ **Don't combine NSAIDs.** For instance, don't take aspirin to help prevent colon cancer, plus ibuprofen for your arthritis. Doubling up poses more damage to the lining in your stomach and small intestine.

▸ **Stop taking aspirin five days before undergoing surgery.** Irish researchers found people's blood began clotting normally again four days after they stopped taking aspirin. You may be able to resume aspirin therapy in as little as two days after surgery, but speak with your doctor first.

Bromelain
Calm colon with a natural enzyme

Pineapples grow from a complex flower. Clusters of tiny flowers form the flower head. As they die, they merge into one large fruit. In fact, each "eye" on a pineapple is a small, dried-up flower.

Christopher Columbus, Sir Walter Raleigh, and other European explorers stumbled upon the fruit in the West Indies in the late 15th

Pineapple plants rarely form seeds. Instead, you can propagate them by rooting the leafy crown of the fruit or a sucker from the plant. The plants need very little water, so they will grow in places with low rainfall. The first fruit should be ready for harvest about 18 months after planting.

century. They introduced it to the rest of the world, where it quickly became a favorite delicacy.

Aside from being tasty treats, pineapples contain bromelain, an enzyme with healing benefits. Bromelain is found in the flesh and stem of fresh pineapples. You can also buy it as a supplement.

This enzyme breaks down protein, so it's often used as an ingredient in meat tenderizers. Nutritionists recommend it as a digestive aid for certain conditions for the same reason.

▸ **Diarrhea.** Bromelain seems to help treat and prevent diarrhea caused by *E. coli*. In one study, a dose of bromelain kept more than half of a group of piglets exposed to *E. coli* from developing diarrhea. Among those not treated with bromelain, none escaped diarrhea. In fact, the more of the enzyme a piglet was given, the better his chances got of avoiding diarrhea.

▸ **Constipation.** Several studies suggest it helps maintain regularity and relieve constipation. In fact, some nutritionists think eating just 4 ounces of pineapple a day may be enough to end constipation. Just remember to discuss chronic or severe constipation with your doctor first.

▸ **Celiac disease.** Experts think bromelain may pick up the slack for people with celiac disease, helping them digest food and giving their digestive system time to heal.

▸ **Ulcerative colitis.** It may do the same for people with ulcerative colitis. Some doctors report bromelain supplements helped people suffering from mild ulcerative colitis by healing the inflamed mucous membrane lining their colons. Animal studies show it may help heal stomach ulcers, as well.

You can get bromelain from eating fresh, not canned or cooked, pineapple, but experts suggest using supplements. They say you may not get enough from food alone for most of these digestive benefits.

4 things you should know about bromelain

Bromelain is no cure-all, but it could offer significant help for serious digestive disorders. If your doctor agrees, try the supplements with a dose of this advice.

▸ *Take bromelain tablets* before or during meals as a digestive aid.

▸ *Aim for 750 to 1,000 milligrams* (mg) of bromelain a day, divided into four doses, for diarrhea caused by *E. coli*.

▸ *Shop for tablets* with at least 1,000 GDUs (gelatin-digesting units). GDUs are one way of measuring supplemental bromelain.

▸ *Limit your dosage* to no more than 2,000 mg a day.

Word to the wise

Bromelain is relatively safe and well-tolerated, with few side effects. Still, some people may be allergic to this enzyme. It may also cause a rapid heartbeat in people with high blood pressure or irritate your stomach if you have ulcers. Take it only as directed. High doses can cause nausea, diarrhea, and other intestinal problems.

Calcium supplements
Vital mineral slashes colon cancer risk

Calcium ranked the third highest selling supplement in the United States in 2002. Although most people take it to prevent osteoporosis, this mineral might offer another important benefit.

Bone up on calcium for healthy intestines, and you might also lower your risk of colon cancer — a common killer that often runs in families. Many studies link calcium intake with a lower risk of colon cancer. The reduction is modest but meaningful, even a small edge could save lives.

All that extra calcium will do you no good if you don't get enough vitamin D. Your body needs vitamin D to put calcium to work. New research shows getting plenty of this vitamin alongside calcium could further lower your risk of colon cancer. Aim for at least 400 International Units (IU) of vitamin D a day from supplements or foods, such as milk, eggs, or salmon. Some calcium supplements also contain vitamin D.

Scientists think calcium protects the lining in your colon from attack by cancer-causing agents, and it may keep the cells lining your intestines from growing out of control.

The mineral seems to prevent precancerous changes in the colon, like the formation of large bowel adenomas or polyps. They don't start out cancerous, but they can become cancerous, and if you have had one, you are likely to develop more.

In a new meta-analysis, researchers looked at the results of three clinical trials involving more than 1,400 people. Each person had had precancerous colon polyps removed, then started taking either calcium supplements or a placebo. On average, those taking calcium had a 20-percent lower risk of recurring polyps than people taking the placebo. Another study from the National Cancer Institute links higher calcium intakes, especially from supplements, to fewer colon polyps.

Calcium from supplements seems to prevent colon cancer better than calcium from food sources. You can choose from three main kinds of calcium supplements.

▸ *Calcium carbonate,* like the antacid Tums, is the cheapest and most convenient source of this mineral. It contains about 40 percent calcium. Unfortunately, it's tough for your gut to absorb and tends to cause the most side effects.

▶ *Calcium citrate* in brands such as Citracal is more expensive but easier to absorb. It only contains 21 percent calcium, less than carbonate, but your body absorbs more of it and with fewer side effects.

▶ *Calcium phosphate* is also more expensive than carbonate and less common. It has about 40 percent calcium.

More isn't always better. Your body has trouble absorbing large doses of this mineral. You benefit more taking smaller doses, around 500 milligrams (mg), throughout the day.

As with all things, calcium has a point of diminishing returns. Experts estimate your risk of colon cancer starts to drop at 700 mg of calcium a day and stops at 1,000 mg a day. Above this dosage, you reap no more reward. Stay within the healthy Adequate Intake (AI) limits and get at least 1,200 mg of calcium each day from food or supplements if you are over age 50.

Never take more than 2,500 mg of calcium daily, including food sources, unless your doctor prescribes otherwise. Too much calcium can interfere with the absorption of other minerals in your body. A few studies suggest very high calcium intakes may increase the risk of prostate cancer, although this link is still unclear.

Word to the wise

Calcium supplements can interact with over-the-counter and prescription medications. Discuss them with your doctor first, especially if you take:

▶ thiazide or similar diuretics

▶ digoxin, a heart medication

▶ tetracycline antibiotics

▶ fluroquinolone antibiotics

▶ levothyroxine, a thyroid hormone

▶ aluminum or magnesium antacids

▶ glucocorticoids, such as prednisone

▶ mineral oil

▶ stimulant laxatives

3 things you should know about calcium supplements

Extra calcium may be good for you, but the gas, bloating, and constipation that sometimes result might encourage you to stop taking them. Try this advice to calm the storm of calcium side effects.

▸ *Take supplements with meals* and drink plenty of fluids during the day.

▸ *Break up large doses* into smaller ones and take them throughout the day. This minimizes discomfort and maximizes the amount of calcium your body absorbs.

▸ *Switch to a different brand if side effects persist.* If they don't improve, discuss your symptoms with your doctor or pharmacist.

Charcoal
Common antidote saves lives

Filtering systems use activated charcoal to take harmful chemicals out of the air or water. Charcoal is good at trapping other organic substances and things like chlorine. But chemicals that are not attracted to carbon will pass right through the filter. Once the charcoal surface is filled, the filter will no longer work, and you need to replace it.

Activated, or medicinal, charcoal is different from the briquettes used to barbecue. It's fine, fluffy, and black with no taste or smell. This charcoal works like a filter in your body and attracts harmful substances. Doctors sometimes use it to treat accidental poisoning.

Manufacturers specially treat this medicinal charcoal with oxygen to open up thousands of tiny pores inside it, making it super adsorbent. ADsorbent is not the same as ABsorbent. Sponges are absorbent. They soak up liquids like water but only hold them temporarily. The water eventually evaporates.

Activated charcoal is adsorbent — it chemically attaches to odors, liquids, and other material, binding to them and trapping them almost permanently.

It has been used as a poisoning antidote for nearly a century because of its amazing ability to adsorb chemicals. Emergency room doctors give liquid charcoal to people who have accidentally poisoned themselves or overdosed on medication. It picks up the chemicals in their digestive tract and carries them safely out of the body.

It also enjoys a simpler use. Doctors sometimes recommend activated charcoal caplets to relieve gas.

Word to the wise

Doctors may give liquid charcoal as a poisoning antidote, but they don't recommend you do it yourself. Studies show most people give the wrong dose when using at home, and the person taking it often vomits it back up.

Don't risk a life by depending on charcoal to treat poisoning. Call your poison control center immediately at 800-222-1222 if you suspect poisoning or an overdose.

3 things you should know about charcoal

Activated charcoal can help relieve gas, but it isn't the answer for everyone. Try this advice if your doctor agrees it might work for you.

▸ *Take between 520 and 975 milligrams* (mg) of activated charcoal in a capsule for gas after meals or as soon as you feel bloated.

▸ *Avoid combining it with medications.* Take it two hours before or one hour after your other medicines.

▸ *Don't take more than 4 grams* (4,000 mg) of activated charcoal in a day. It can clump in your intestines and cause serious problems.

Chewing gum
Simple way to stick it to heartburn

Chewing gum might help you recover from colon surgery. According to recent research, people who chewed gum after elective colon surgery left the hospital sooner. All 102 participants in the study had undergone removal of a portion of the colon, either conventional surgery or the less-invasive laparoscopic version. In addition, half the patients had the usual recovery diet, while the others also got chewing gum at meal times. Gum chewers who had laparoscopic surgery got out of the hospital one day sooner than those who went gum-free. Because surgery usually stills the digestive system for awhile, scientists think chewing gum might help the digestive tract restart itself sooner.

Scientific studies show smacking on a stick of gum could relieve heartburn as well as, or better than, antacids. Chewing regular or sugar-free gum stimulates the flow of saliva, which contains healing factors the body produces to help repair damage in the digestive tract, plus natural antacids. This extra spit neutralizes the acid that has leaked into your esophagus, the cause of that uncomfortable, burning feeling, and washes it back down to your stomach.

A small but significant clinical trial shows chewing a stick of gum after meals may counteract acid reflux. Researchers studied 12 people with gastroesophageal reflux disease (GERD) and 24 people without GERD. Chewing gum for an hour after eating lowered the amount of acid in the esophagus of GERD sufferers for three hours. Since acid reflux usually occurs within three hours of eating, these experts say gum lasts long enough to manage after-meal reflux.

If that sounds good, get ready for even more relief. A few manufacturers now make gum containing an antacid such as calcium carbonate, the active ingredient in Tums. This combines the power of an antacid tablet with your body's own saliva, boosting gum's power to put out the flames.

In fact, antacid gum may relieve heartburn faster and for a longer time than regular gum or antacid alone. Experts at the Oklahoma Foundation for Digestive Research gave volunteers a high-dose antacid gum, low-dose antacid gum, chewable antacid tablet, or placebo.

Word to the wise

Skip spearmint- or peppermint-flavored gum if you are chewing to battle heartburn. They can actually make reflux worse. Peppermint, in particular, relaxes the lower ring muscle in your esophagus, allowing acid to creep up from your stomach.

Both the high- and low-dose gums soothed heartburn and neutralized acid in the esophagus better than placebo. They eased discomfort for at least two hours after meals, and both worked faster and provided longer-lasting relief than the antacid tablet alone.

3 things you should know about chewing gum

If you suffer from heartburn or GERD, grab a stick and start chewing for quick relief.

▸ *Chew regular gum for 30 to 60 minutes after a meal* or when heartburn sets in.

▸ *Opt for sugar-free gum to prevent cavities,* but avoid gum made with artificial sweeteners if they give you digestive problems. Sorbitol, for instance, can cause gas, bloating, and diarrhea.

▸ *Look for Chooz, an antacid gum,* at your local pharmacy. If they don't carry it, ask them to order it for you, or buy it on the Internet.

Laxatives
Help for sluggish bowels

Doctors usually recommend laxatives for occasional or chronic constipation, as well as emptying the bowels before colonoscopy, X-rays of the digestive tract, and other procedures. When used properly, laxatives can safely and effectively treat constipation.

Constipation is one of the most common gastrointestinal complaints in Western countries. People in the United States make 2.5 million doctor visits each year for constipation and spend hundreds of millions of dollars on laxatives.

But the best, cheapest, and simplest solution by far is to load up your plate with more high-fiber foods. In fact, bulking agents — some of the most common laxatives — are made of fiber. You could get the same effect just eating more fibrous foods every day, including fresh vegetables, fruits, bran, beans, and whole grains. Getting plenty of liquids and regular exercise will also keep your bowels moving smoothly. You can read about the many other health benefits of fiber in the *Fiber* section in Chapter 4.

Your doctor may still recommend laxatives in addition to dietary and lifestyle changes. Generally, you can choose from five kinds of laxative.

▸ *Bulking agents.* Psyllium (Metamucil), methylcellulose (Citrucel), calcium polycarbophil (Fibercon), bran, flaxseed, and glucomann absorb water in the intestines, making the stool softer and easier to move. They also add bulk, which triggers bowel contractions.

Bulk laxatives are one of the safest to help you get regular, and you can take them to treat, as well as prevent, chronic constipation. Side effects include gas and bloating.

▸ *Stool softeners.* Docusate (Colase, Surfak) contains detergents that enable the stool to absorb and hold more water. This softens them and adds bulk, which triggers contractions in your large intestine.

Stool softeners work best for people who need to avoid straining during bowel movements, such as those with hemorrhoids or who have recently had surgery. People sometimes experience nausea with these laxatives, especially when taking the liquid form.

▶ **Osmotics.** These laxatives contain lactulose, sodium phosphate, sorbitol, or magnesium salts, such as magnesium hydroxide and magnesium citrate. These salts and sugars pull water into the large intestine, loosening and softening the stool. The water also stretches the large intestine, which triggers bowel contractions.

Osmotics are better at treating constipation than preventing it. Doctors often prescribe them as preparation for X-rays of the digestive tract or colonoscopies. They work in about three hours. However, they may cause people with kidney disease or heart failure to retain excessive fluid. Magnesium- and phosphate-containing osmotics are especially dangerous to people with kidney failure. Those made with lactose or sorbitol can cause cramps and gas.

▶ **Stimulants.** Doctors often prescribe these before surgery and other procedures to empty the large intestine. They often contain ingredients, such as senna or cascara, that irritate the

Word to the wise

Watch for signs of magnesium overdose. Many laxatives, such as Milk of Magnesia, contain magnesium salts because they work fast, but too much can be toxic. Call a doctor immediately if you experience light-headedness, low blood pressure, muscle weakness, confusion, heart rhythm abnormalities, nausea, or vomiting.

People with kidney problems, in particular, should avoid magnesium laxatives. The American College of Gastroenterology recommends only using them in special, severe cases of constipation, and only for short periods.

walls of your intestines, making them contract and move the stool along. Unfortunately, stimulants may also cause cramps and diarrhea.

Take them orally, and you will usually have a semisolid bowel movement in six to eight hours. Suppositories work in 15 to 60 minutes. Stimulant laxatives include cascara, senna (Senekot, Fletcher's Castoria), castor oil, bisacodyl (Dulcolax, Ex-lax), and sennosides (Correctol).

▸ **Lubricants.** Products like mineral oil grease the stool so it slips more easily through the intestines. Mineral oil has been used for many years, but beware — it can cause your body to fail to absorb vitamins and calcium. It also may interfere with drugs aimed at preventing blood clots. If you take anticoagulants, talk with your doctor before using mineral oil.

While psyllium's soluble fiber adds bulk to the stool, it can clog you up if not taken with plenty of water or balanced with bran and other insoluble fiber. Keep this in mind when using a psyllium product.

Experts have long believed taking stimulant laxatives regularly for long periods of time could lead to dependence, rebound constipation, and even permanent colon damage.

But now scientists are taking a second look. A new review published by the American College of Gastroenterology, the foremost authority on digestive disorders, says long-term use of stimulant laxatives does not cause these problems if taken in the recommended doses. However, they note some people do abuse laxatives, which can lead to serious health problems.

Health professionals will have to consider the new findings. Meanwhile, they advise only using stimulant laxatives for short periods of time. If you need them for more than a week, take them only every third day, and only under your doctor's supervision.

Many commercial laxatives contain more than one ingredient, combining, for instance, a stool softener and a stimulant laxative.

Aloe juice gets things moving

You may already know aloe is good for your skin, but did you know it's been curing digestive dilemmas for centuries?

Aloe gel softens skin. Aloe juice, on the other hand, helps relieve constipation and hemorrhoids. The gel and juice come from the same plant but different parts of the leaf.

People have used the bitter, yellow aloe juice as a laxative for roughly 1,800 years. It contains anthraquinones called aloins A and B. When you swallow aloe juice, these aloins pass through to your colon. Intestinal bacteria break them down into metabolites, which stimulate your gastrointestinal tract.

That stimulation speeds up the movement through your bowel, so less water gets absorbed from the stool. More movement and softer stool mean less constipation, which may, in turn, ease hemorrhoids.

▸ Aloe juice comes in liquid form or dried, as a resin. But don't use aloe extract or reconstituted aloe, made from powdered or liquid concentrate. Most of the time, they are too diluted.

▸ Buy a product with at least 70-percent aloe. If a product doesn't list percentages on the label, read the ingredients. Aloe vera should be near the top of the list. If not, don't bother buying the product.

▸ Don't take aloe for more than two weeks. You may become dependent on it. And follow the directions carefully — an overdose can cause severe diarrhea.

▸ Get plenty of fluids and electrolytes, especially potassium, while taking aloe juice. Broths, soups, fruit juices, fruits, clear soda, and gelatin are good choices

Combination products do not necessarily work better than single ingredients, and they tend to cause more side effects.

You can buy most laxatives over the counter without a prescription, but don't treat yourself long-term with them. Seek out real, safe relief by speaking with your doctor about persistent constipation. A serious health problem could be causing it, and in some cases, drug side effects are to blame. Your doctor can properly diagnose the problem and recommend an occasional laxative to offset drug side effects.

14 things you should know about laxatives

So many options, so much advice. Here's a guide to help you decide which laxative is right for you and how to get the most benefit.

▸ **Drink plenty of fluids** with bulk-forming laxatives, and skip them if you have trouble swallowing. They can get stuck in your esophagus.

▸ **Begin by taking small amounts** of bulking agents and gradually increase your dosage, following the directions on the label, until you have regular bowel movements.

▸ **Discuss bulk laxatives with your doctor** as they may prevent your body from absorbing some medications. Diabetics, in particular, should avoid them.

▸ **Take liquid stool softeners with milk or fruit juice** to improve the taste.

▸ **Wash down osmotics with 8 ounces of cold water** or fruit juice, and then follow up with a second glass. These laxatives need plenty of fluid to work well.

▸ **Skip stimulant laxatives,** such as senna, if you have diverticulosis because they can irritate your colon. Instead, look to natural softeners, like prunes, prune juice, and psyllium.

▸ **Only take senna laxatives short-term** for occasional constipation, and do not take them more than two weeks without the advice of your doctor. Also, avoid using them if you take thiazide diuretics or adrenocorticosteroids.

▸ **Don't take castor oil at bedtime** because it works faster than most other laxatives. And don't use it regularly to treat constipation. Its action may be too strong for safe regular use.

▸ **Kill the bad taste of castor oil** by refrigerating it, and then mix it with cold orange juice just before drinking.

▸ **Don't crush or chew bisacodyl tablets,** and avoid taking them within an hour of drinking milk or using antacids.

▸ **Check with your doctor or pharmacist** before trying stimulant laxatives if you are on a low-sugar, low-sodium, or low-calorie diet. Some contain large amounts of salt, sugar, or carbohydrates.

▸ **Wait at least two hours after meals** before taking mineral oil to minimize its interference with your body's absorption of nutrients.

▸ **Don't take mineral oil for long periods of time.** It can build up within body tissue and lead to other health problems.

▸ **Never give mineral oil to someone who is bedridden** or has trouble swallowing. Inhaling drops of it can cause pneumonia.

Nicotine patch
Surprising help for ulcerative colitis

Everyone knows nicotine is generally bad for you. An addictive drug, it raises your risk for cancer and ulcers, worsens other digestive problems, and suppresses your immune system. But scientists say it may help ease the symptoms of ulcerative colitis (UC).

Nonsmokers have almost three times the risk of developing UC as smokers, while the more heavily people smoke, the smaller their chance of getting UC. Of course, the risks of smoking far outweigh potential benefits, so scientists are seeking other ways to get the advantage of nicotine without the harm. Adhesive skin patches that deliver a constant dose of nicotine into the bloodstream could play a role.

Some evidence suggests UC develops from a malfunction in your immune system. Nicotine may suppress the immune system, helping put a lid on this condition. The drug also boosts the amount of mucus made in your colon, thickening the protective lining, and it seems to soothe and prevent colon inflammation by squelching the production of prostaglandins, chemicals that cause inflammation.

In one clinical trial, twice as many people with ulcerative colitis went into remission after six weeks on a nicotine patch as did on a placebo. The patch users also saw their UC symptoms improve and had fewer bowel movements, as well as less abdominal pain and urgency.

The people in this study continued taking their regular UC medications while on the nicotine patch. But another clinical trial testing the patch on its own found it did not prevent relapse any more than the placebo. A third study found the patch was not as effective as prednisone in improving UC. Only 30 percent of people improved using the nicotine patch, compared to 60 percent taking prednisone. However, taking prednisone for long periods causes very serious side effects.

The key seems to lie in using nicotine patches as a co-therapy, while taking traditional UC medications, experts say. In this way, the patches may help maintain remission and relieve symptoms during flare-ups. Doctors do not recommend treating UC with nicotine alone since studies so far have shown it doesn't work as well as with combined therapy.

Nicotine patches also carry side effects, such as rash, nausea, and lightheadedness, and many people do not tolerate them well. However, ulcerative colitis is such a serious

Word to the wise

Experts say nicotine, not just cigarettes, can lead to serious health problems. Nicotine increases your risk of developing a stomach ulcer or suffering a relapse, and it delays the healing of ulcers. It also promotes cancer — even the patch may raise your risk of this deadly disease. Weigh the pros and cons of the nicotine patch with your doctor before using it to treat ulcerative colitis.

condition that the risk of side effects from nicotine may be a small price to pay for possible remission. Just remember — taking nicotine in any form for this condition is still an experimental and controversial treatment.

2 things you should know about the nicotine patch

Studies suggest the nicotine patch may help people suffering with UC, but before you try it, talk with your doctor — and keep these things in mind.

▶ *Use a patch delivering 15 milligrams* (mg) of nicotine daily.

▶ *Consider trying nicotine gum* if you don't like the patch. Some UC studies have found similar success with the gum.

Also, remember to keep taking your regular medicine for UC. Research shows the patch only helps if taken along with traditional UC medications.

Nicotine is a highly addictive drug, according to the National Institutes of Health. It has effects similar to cocaine, heroin, and marijuana, increasing the levels of the brain chemical dopamine, which affects the pleasure centers in the brain.

Pig whipworm egg therapy
Experimental treatment foils Crohn's

Over 70 percent of people with active Crohn's disease went into remission after six months of pig whipworm egg therapy, according to a University of Iowa study. Pig whipworm eggs don't cause a lasting infection in humans. They are expelled within a day or two without causing significant symptoms of parasite infection. Although FDA approval requires much larger trials, these astonishing results might mean a brighter future for the many people who live with Crohn's disease.

The researchers behind this doctor-formulated preparation suggest it might reset the faulty immune system response that causes symptoms of inflammatory bowel disease. Not only has this therapy shown promise with Crohn's disease, and studies also suggest it may ease ulcerative colitis symptoms in some people. However, the benefit in treating ulcerative colitis may not be as great as the dramatic remissions experienced by many people with Crohn's.

Fewer people might have Crohn's disease if more of them had had intestinal parasites as children when their immune systems were developing. At least that's the "hygiene theory" that inspired University of Iowa gastroenterologist Joel Weinstock and his colleagues to create pig whipworm egg therapy. The scientists point out that Crohn's is rare in parts of the world where intestinal parasites are common. In fact, Crohn's has been on the rise in developed countries for the last 50 years as rates of intestinal parasite cases have plummeted.

A 12-week trial compared 30 ulcerative colitis sufferers on pig whipworm egg therapy to 24 ulcerative colitis sufferers on placebo. While the therapy didn't appear to trigger remission of symptoms any better than the placebo, 43 percent of the study participants on pig whipworm egg therapy reported symptom improvement compared to 16 percent of the participants who took a placebo.

Although participants in both the Crohn's and ulcerative colitis studies did not stop taking their regular medicines when they began pig whipworm egg therapy, no one reported any drug interactions. Almost no side effects from the therapy were reported either.

Participants in both studies took doses of 2,500 pig whipworm eggs. But those in the Crohn's study took their dose every three weeks, while those with ulcerative colitis took it every two weeks. However, the

Crohn's study ran for six months —
twice as long as the ulcerative colitis
study. The Crohn's study was smaller and lacked a control group, but it
ran longer and the results were
more promising.

The authors of these studies point
out that symptoms of inflammatory
bowel diseases apparently are
caused by an overactive immune
reaction. Crohn's symptoms may be
triggered by overactive immune cells
called TH1, while ulcerative colitis
symptoms could be the fault of TH2
immune cells. Pig whipworm eggs

mainly seem to stifle the activity of TH1 cells. But they may also help
keep TH2 cells from being quite so rambunctious.

The researchers also emphasize that these particular whipworms
aren't going to give you worms because they don't infect humans at
this stage. In fact, that's why they chose the pig whipworm. Pig
whipworms can survive just long enough in your gut to rein in overactive factors in the immune system, probably because they're related
to the Trichuris trichiura intestinal worm that can infect humans. But
these are pig whipworms — Trichuris suis. They need some time in
the dirt before they can infect a host.

Although pig whipworm egg therapy appears to be more effective
for Crohn's than ulcerative colitis, more research is needed to be sure.
Stay tuned to find out whether this unusual new therapy can be
effective and safe over the long term.

2 things you should know about pig whipworm egg therapy

Pig whipworm egg therapy is so new it isn't widely available. Here
are two things to keep in mind if you are interested in trying it.

▸ **Get more information.** The FDA has not approved this therapy, but you can order a pig whipworm egg therapy product from Germany with a doctor's help, if he approves. An order must include a letter from a licensed doctor and a letter from the patient as the receiver. The letters must include the patient's address and telephone number, as well as the doctor's. For more details, visit the Ovamed Web site at *www.ovamed.de* or e-mail them at info@ovamed.de.

For more information

Ovamed GmbH
Kiebitzhörn 33-35
22885 Barsbüttel
Germany

▸ **Follow the directions carefully.** Have juice or a sports drink, like Gatorade, on hand if you try the pig whipworm egg therapy product called TSO. The product instructions recommend you dilute TSO with drinks like these instead of alcoholic beverages or hot drinks.

Therapeutic massage
Turn your back on stress-induced flare-ups

A therapeutic massage could be just what you need. Not only can it melt stress away, but it may also help any digestive condition or illness that can be triggered by stress or aggravated by it. Therapeutic massage might also take the flames out of digestive flare-ups or even prevent them from happening at all. Scientists even suggest it shows promise as a remedy for constipation.

Massages offer two kinds of help. First, massage can muzzle stomach-twisting stress. Science shows this stress can contribute to indigestion, heartburn, IBS symptoms, IBD flare-ups, and more. Stress can even trigger a surprise round of diarrhea.

And a study supported by the National Institute of Mental Health found that massage therapy eased depression and anxiety and reduced levels of stress hormones, like cortisol. Massage also stimulates your brain to produce more endorphins, chemicals that help block pain and increase your sense of well-being.

But massage may have an even more direct effect on your digestive system. In a small study, some people who had colon surgery received a special stomach massage. Starting the second day after surgery, those who got the special massage had less pain and needed fewer painkillers than those who didn't.

Some natural healers recommend massaging your lower stomach in a clockwise motion to ease constipation. Little research has been done to verify this, but scientists think stomach massage may show promise for chronic constipation.

When most people think of massage, they picture Swedish massage with its long strokes and kneading, but other kinds of massage are available, too. For example, deep tissue massage uses heavier pressure to work deeper layers of muscle, while sports massage is geared toward helping athletes.

If you consider massage an unnecessary luxury, you may want to see what your doctor says. Fifty-four percent of primary care doctors and family practitioners surveyed said they would encourage their patients to consider massage therapy to supplement medical treatment.

You may have considered trying massage in the past but hesitated because of concern about quacks or seedy massage parlors. But avoiding these problems is a lot easier than in the past. At least 35 states either regulate massage therapists or require them to be licensed. You're even more likely to find a good massage therapist if your doctor can recommend one.

A typical massage session lasts about an hour. You'll undress either partially or completely. But you'll be draped with a towel or sheet to preserve modesty and keep you warm during the massage. The price of a single table massage ranges between $50 and $85.

You may prefer to try a seated or chair massage, which does not require you to undress. Seated massages are done in special massage chairs and usually last 30 minutes or less.

7 things you should know about therapeutic massage

Knowledge and preparation will ensure you have a relaxing, comfortable experience.

▸ *Find a trained and qualified massage therapist* to avoid mishaps. Try calling the American Massage Therapy Association at 888-843-2682, or visit its Web site at *www.amtamassage.org,* and click on Find a Massage Therapist.

Word to the wise

Check with your doctor before scheduling a massage if you have a heart condition. Avoid massage if you have a fever, infectious skin disease, rash, abdominal hernia, cancer, or circulation problems, like phlebitis, blood clots, or varicose veins. Don't allow the therapist to massage bruised, inflamed, or infected areas, recent fractures, or sprains. And don't get a massage immediately after surgery.

▸ *Wear loose, comfortable clothes.* Most people remove all or part of their clothing for the massage. But if you prefer not to, remember the therapist needs to be able to reach the areas you want worked on.

▸ *Do not eat right before a massage session.* Don't allow massage in your stomach area for at least two hours after eating.

▸ *Remove any jewelry* that might get in the way of your massage.

▸ *Tell your therapist* if you are allergic to any oils, lotions, or their ingredients. Some massage therapists can use powder in place of oil.

▸ *Get off the table slowly* if you are dizzy after the massage.

▸ *Drink extra water* after your session.

YOU WANT TO FIND OUT WHAT'S TROUBLING YOU, but you're worried about diagnostic tests and doctor visits. Now you can learn how to determine if a test is appropriate, what to expect, and how to discover steps that may help you gain more control over your health.

CHAPTER 7

Medical tests to diagnose digestive diseases

What happens in a medical exam makes more sense when you realize your doctor is like a detective. He takes the clues he gets from you and uses them to uncover the health problem that's bothering you. Here's how you can help.

▸ Start keeping a food and symptom diary as soon as you know you'll be going to the doctor. Track what you eat and everything about your symptoms, including when they happen, what they're like, and what relieves them.

▸ Bring a bag of all the prescription and over-the-counter medicines and supplements you take. If you decide to make a list instead, be sure to include the name of the medicine and the dosage.

▸ Be ready to give very specific descriptions of pain you experience, including what kind it is, how intense, how often you have it and how long, other symptoms that go with it, and what seems to help, if anything.

▸ Be prepared to give details about your medical history. Make sure your doctor has access to all your medical records.

Your doctor can also find clues from your weight, blood pressure, temperature, and physical appearance. Further clues come from the questions he asks you about your symptoms, eating habits, and activities.

During the physical exam, your doctor may check more than just your abdominal area. That's because clues to digestive ills can lurk in many places. You can also expect him to:

▸ look in your mouth and listen to your chest with a stethoscope if he suspects a problem with your esophagus.

▸ check your abdomen from different angles to look for swelling or signs of trouble in a particular part of your digestive system.

▸ listen to your stomach with a stethoscope to hear any sounds that may point to a particular problem.

- tap across your stomach area to check the size of your liver and spleen and detect any swelling that might be a symptom of too much fluid or gas.

- press on your abdominal area gently to check for tenderness, signs of inflammation or infection, abnormal masses, enlarged organs, hardened stool, or other signs of trouble.

- search for enlarged lymph glands by feeling your neck, under your arms, and other areas.

- check your anus and surrounding area for inflammation or other signs of problems.

- perform a digital rectal exam with a lubricated, gloved finger to inspect for hemorrhoids or anal fissures.

After the exam, your doctor may order diagnostic tests. Learning more about a test can make it less frightening because you'll know what to expect. For example, some diagnostic scanners make loud noises or require you to fit into a tight space. Fortunately, expected loud noises are less likely to startle you, and mild sedatives are available if you have claustrophobia or fear of being confined.

According to a recent report by The Wall Street Journal, some doctors may be making extra money when they order a test. If a doctor can find a testing lab that charges less than the reimbursement amount he'll get from insurance, he can make a profit when the reimbursement payment comes in. As long as the insurance company doesn't discover that the test was done "on the cheap" by an outside lab, it's easy money. The report points out that this might tempt a doctor to order more tests than you really need.

You might discover that you shouldn't take the test right now. The test may have "contraindications," meaning that some people can't take this test or can only do so under specific conditions. For example, some people can never take a particular test because of a health problem, pacemaker or other implant, or other reasons. Others may merely need to delay the test temporarily until they've recovered from a surgery, illness, or the effects of another test.

Some tests can't determine exactly what's wrong. Instead, they help your doctor narrow down the list of possible problems. Other tests have a high rate of false positives. If the test doesn't give specific answers or has a high rate of false positives, you usually need more tests. Sometimes you might be better off if you started with a different test in the first place.

Even worse, some tests have a high rate of false negatives. That means the test will tell you that you don't have a problem, even though you do.

Learning about a test might mean you avoid having to take it twice. Why? Because things you do can affect the results of a test. Moving too much during a scan might make the pictures too blurred to be useful. In addition, you might accidentally eat something or do something that could cause a false positive or false negative.

You just found out that your test results are "abnormal." Before you worry, discuss these questions with your doctor.

▶ Did I have a list of things to do before the test? A list of things to avoid? Did I follow those instructions carefully?

▶ Are the test results abnormal enough to be a real concern?

▶ Do I have a habit, health condition, or other circumstance that could skew the test results?

On top of all that, some tests can be less safe or less accurate when an inexperienced or poorly trained person is running the test equipment or interpreting the results.

Even a mix-up in paperwork or a computer glitch can affect your test. Sometimes the most dedicated and caring member of a medical staff can make an honest mistake that leads to someone receiving the wrong test. Nearly all tests have risks. Your best bet is to find out the risks and benefits of taking the test, as well as the hazards of avoiding the test.

In his book, *The Last Well Person*, medical school professor Nortin M. Hadler, M.D., questions whether screening tests, like colonoscopy, are right for everyone, especially for those who don't have symptoms of disease, partly because of the risks involved. Some health experts question whether every test ordered is genuinely necessary. In fact, your doctor may feel he has no choice but to order some tests, whether you need them or not. Consequently, if he is ever sued for malpractice, he can produce a record of the tests he ordered to show that he did everything possible to make sure the diagnosis was right.

So what can you do when your doctor wants to do a test? Ask questions. Use these examples to guide you.

▶ What is the purpose of the test?

▶ How accurate is the test? What are the rates of false positives and false negatives?

▶ What are the risks of this test? Do the benefits outweigh the risks?

▶ What health issues, medicines, or past surgeries might make this test unsafe for me?

▶ What information will you look for in the test results? Is there another safer, cheaper, or less painful way to find that out?

▶ When was the last time the test equipment was checked for safety and accuracy?

▶ Are side effects possible from dye, barium, or other chemicals used during the test? How long should these last? Will I be exposed to radiation? Is there protection I can wear?

▶ How much does the test cost? Will my insurance company cover the test?

And right before you take a test, ask for whom the test was ordered. Make sure you get the test that's meant for you. Also, ask your doctor if he has any handouts or other information that can tell you more about the test.

The remainder of this chapter is chock full of information about tests for digestive system problems. Start reading so you can learn valuable information that can help you stay on top of your health.

Blood tests

Blood tests are usually low-risk and cheaper than many other tests. They can help diagnose some problems and rule out others. Just remember that prescription and over-the-counter drugs and supplements can interfere with blood test results, so tell your doctor about the drugs and supplements you take.

Here are some of the blood tests doctors often use to diagnose digestive problems.

Complete blood count. This test provides information about the properties of your blood, including red blood cell count and white blood cell count. Lowered red blood cell count (anemia) may be a symptom of bleeding in the colon, rectum, stomach, or elsewhere in your body. Increased white blood cell count may mean you have inflammation or infection somewhere in your body.

Food sensitivity tests. Blood tests for antibodies with names like IgG4, IgE, IgA, and IgM can help spot food sensitivities. You may hear this test called ELISA (Enzyme-Linked Immunosorbent Assay.)

Celiac disease test. Tests for allergies won't detect celiac disease. Instead, doctors often use tests that check for other antibodies, like the endomysial antibody and tissue transglutaminase antibody tests. Although the test called the gliadin antibody test has also been used, this test is less accurate. Tests on saliva or stool for antibodies are probably weak substitutes for the blood test. A biopsy that can be taken during a colonoscopy is the most definitive test for celiac disease.

Blood tests for pancreatitis. Amylase and lipase are digestive enzymes formed in the pancreas. Although these enzymes show up in your bloodstream when you're healthy, their amounts triple during acute pancreatitis. Enzyme tests like these may not be sensitive enough for chronic pancreatitis, so your doctor may order a test called the secretin stimulation test if he suspects chronic pancreatitis, especially if you're having trouble absorbing some nutrients.

Your doctor may also order blood tests that check for electrolytes, parasites, or bacterial infections. Electrolyte tests check for sodium, potassium, chloride, and carbon dioxide. Unusual levels of these can give clues to what's wrong. A blood test may also be one of the tests your doctor uses to check for *H. pylori*, the bacterium that causes ulcers and may lead to stomach cancer. Blood tests can also reveal an elevated erythrocyte sedimentation rate (ESR), a sign of inflammation.

Liver function tests

These blood tests check how well your liver is functioning. Other than the discomfort of having blood drawn, this is an easy test for both you and your wallet.

Abnormal amounts of several normally occurring substances in the blood may signal problems in your liver or related organs. Depending on which substances are checked, the blood test can help diagnose or rule out conditions like these:

▸ obstruction of the bile ducts

▸ cirrhosis of the liver

▸ malnutrition

▸ vitamin D deficiency

▸ pernicious anemia

▸ hepatitis

Ask your doctor for detailed instructions about how to prepare for the test. Even if you are healthy, factors like obesity, drinking alcohol, and taking vitamin supplements, prescription drugs, or over-the-counter medicine can change the current amount of one or more liver-related chemicals.

Although this test is simple, it may not be the only test you need for a diagnosis. On a scale of 1 to 7 where 7 is the most expensive, this test rates a 1.

Stool test

Your stool contains food residue, water, bacteria, cells, mucus, and other body waste. Some of these can guide your doctor toward a diagnosis. That's why stool tests are important. These tests are done either at your doctor's office or at home.

For at-home stool tests, your doctor gives you a kit and instructions on how to collect stool or samples from stool. You may also be given instructions on what to avoid or do during the days before the test starts. In some cases, you may have to take a laxative before the testing begins. Usually the stools must be collected for several days and then returned to your doctor's office or sent to a lab.

Stool tests can check for bacteria, parasites, blood, fat, nutrient absorption, and pancreatic enzymes. These, in turn, can help rule out or diagnose infections, parasites, Crohn's disease, chronic pancreatitis, food poisoning, or ulcerative colitis.

Urine tests

Urine tests are easy and painless because you merely "fill the cup" and hand it off for analysis. Doctors use some urine tests to help make a diagnosis or narrow the possibilities down to a short list. Your doctor may order a urine test to check for infection, a kidney stone, or the source of food poisoning.

If your doctor suspects advanced pancreatitis, he may use a low-cost urine test called the bentiromide test. You must have normal kidney function, and your intestines must be able to absorb nutrients normally for this test to work. If you have chronic pancreatitis, you'll have low levels of a compound called para-aminobenzoic acid (PABA) in your urine.

Lactose intolerance test

Lactose is a sugar naturally found in milk and other dairy products. If you don't make enough lactase, the enzyme you need to digest lactose, it could be causing uncomfortable digestive symptoms, like nausea, pain, gas, and diarrhea.

If you think you are lactose intolerant, try this self-test. Eliminate all dairy products from your diet for at least 10 days. Read labels thoroughly to make sure no lactose sneaks in through packaged foods, pasta, canned goods, drinks, or other foods. Even if a label doesn't list milk or yogurt, you may find these dairy by-products — casein, sodium caseinate, dry milk solids, and whey — in lots of foods.

If you're not sure whether something contains lactose, don't eat it. And keep in mind that about 20 percent of all prescription drugs and 6 percent of all over-the-counter products contain lactose. If your symptoms get better after 10 days or so, treat yourself to one dairy food or drink. If your symptoms return, you may be lactose intolerant. Talk with your doctor about your self-test, especially if it doesn't give you clear results.

A blood test or breath test, or both, may help you find out whether lactose intolerance is making you miserable. The amount of glucose in your blood or hydrogen in your breath can show whether you can digest lactose.

Before the test. Avoid food, drink, smoking, and heavy exercise for eight hours before the blood or breath test. Tell your doctor about all medicines and supplements you take.

Word to the wise

If you have diabetes, your blood test results may say you're not lactose intolerant, even though you really are. This happens because the blood test results can be affected by your blood sugar. Tell your doctor that you have diabetes and ask how you can avoid a false-positive result.

What to expect. A lab technician will draw a blood sample from your arm. Then you will drink a lactose-infused solution. You'll have three more blood samples taken — one 30 minutes after the drink, another one hour after, and a third at two hours. You may also be asked to breathe out into a special device, which measures the amount of hydrogen in your breath. If you have lactose intolerance, the test will probably cause you to have the same symptoms as when you drink milk or eat dairy products.

After the test. You can go back to your normal diet, medications, and activities.

Advantages and disadvantages. Other than possible lactose intolerance symptoms, the test has no side effects or risks. However, some people may still need other tests in addition to these. On a cost scale of 1 to 7 where 7 is the most expensive, this test rates a 3.

Tests for *H. pylori*

Helicobacter pylori (*H. pylori*) is a spiral-shaped bacterium that can lurk in your stomach. It's the troublemaker behind most peptic ulcers, which form in your stomach or small intestine, and it raises your risk of stomach cancer. You also need to know whether you have *H. pylori* because ulcers from *H. pylori* are treated differently than ulcers from other causes.

Four tests are used to detect *H. Pylori* — a blood test, breath test, stool test, and tissue test, which uses a tissue sample, or biopsy, removed with an endoscope.

The blood test is the most common. It detects antibodies to *H. pylori* bacteria. However, blood tests aren't used after an ulcer has been treated with antibiotics because your blood can test positive years after *H. pylori* has been wiped out.

Neither the breath test nor the stool test has that problem. You can take the urea breath test at your doctor's office. You just drink a liquid that contains a special carbon atom. If *H. pylori* is present, it breaks down the urea, setting the carbon free. The blood carries the carbon to your lungs, where it's exhaled.

The stool test is called the *H. pylori* stool antigen test. Studies have shown that this accurately detects *H. pylori*. It's used not only for diagnosis but to help determine whether antibiotics got rid of *H. pylori*.

Blood, breath, and stool tests are often done to see if an upper endoscopy with biopsy should be done. Testing of the biopsy tissue can give the most definitive diagnosis of *H. pylori*.

CT scan

A CT scan painlessly builds a three-dimensional picture of your internal organs. It's like a computerized super X-ray. Instead of taking just one picture, the X-ray machine rotates around you to get pictures from all sides. A computer assembles these images into a cross section of your organs — like one slice from a loaf of bread. That shows the potential problem area in incredible detail from every angle.

Why be tested. A CT scan may be used to diagnose or rule out the following problems:

- causes of abdominal pain, such as an inflamed colon, diverticulitis, appendicitis, infection, or an abscess (a fluid-filled membrane) in your abdomen
- bowel obstruction
- pancreatitis
- gallstones
- cancer

Before the test. Tell your doctor and the CT technologist these things before a scan:

- ▶ what allergies you have, especially reactions to drugs or iodine

- ▶ whether you have a history of diabetes, asthma, heart conditions, kidney problems, or thyroid conditions

- ▶ if you are claustrophobic

- ▶ which medicines you take, especially if you take warfarin or another anticoagulant (blood thinner) drug

You may be told to avoid eating and drinking for an hour or longer before the scan. However, be sure to drink as much water as possible before this fasting period begins.

Plan to remove and store jewelry and other metal-containing items, like clothing with zippers, because metal can interfere with the scan.

What to expect. The CT technologist may ask you to swallow a contrast material, a liquid that makes your stomach, small intestine, and colon easier to see on X-rays. Sometimes the contrast material is given by enema or injection instead. Normal side effects include nausea, headache, and feeling flushed. But tell the technologist immediately if you feel itchy or short of breath. Those may be signs of an allergic reaction.

The technologist will position you on a table that can move in and out of the scanner, as well as up and down. You'll be alone in the room during the scan, but the technologist can see and hear you. She will tell you when each scan sequence is about to begin and how long it will last. She may even ask you to hold your breath for a few seconds. Remain as still as possible throughout the sequence, or you'll blur the image. Try not to be startled by the

A new kind of CT scanner is the helical or spiral scanner. This speedy test can slash the amount of time it takes to complete a scan. High-speed scanners are also used for CT portography, a test that can find tiny liver tumors.

scanner's clicking and whirring. A CT scan usually takes between five minutes and an hour.

Side effects and risks. People with allergies to iodine or shellfish may have an allergic reaction to the contrast dye if it is iodine based. The contrast dye may raise the risk of renal failure in older adults who have either chronic dehydration or kidney impairment. People with claustrophobia may have trouble in tube-shaped CT scanners. Although the levels of radiation during the scan are low, you get more radiation than you would with a simple X-ray. However, CT scans are monitored and regulated so you get the bare minimum of radiation needed to generate the image.

After the test. Most CT scans allow you to get back to normal eating and drinking immediately afterward. But drink plenty of clear liquids to help flush the dye out of your system. Call your doctor if you get hives, rash, or itching within a few hours of completing the test. This could be an allergic reaction to the contrast dye.

Advantages and disadvantages. Pictures from the scan include enough quality and detail to spot problems as small as an inch across. What's more, CT scans make muscles and other soft tissues show up better than regular X-rays. CT scan pictures are also clearer than ultrasound pictures. While the risk from a single CT scan isn't very high, regularly repeated scans might possibly allow radiation to accumulate enough to be a concern. The scan can be uncomfortable and lengthy, and it may find a problem without giving you a final diagnosis. People over 300 pounds may not be able to take this test. On a cost scale of 1 to 7 where 7 is the most expensive, this test rates a 5.

Barium swallow

This test helps your doctor diagnose problems in your esophagus, stomach, and duodenum — the first part of the small intestine. It uses X-rays and barium, a liquid contrast dye that helps organs show up more clearly on X-rays, to examine your digestive tract for diseases and malfunctions.

Why be tested. The barium swallow may be used to diagnose or rule out problems like these:

▸ dysphagia or difficulty swallowing

▸ ulcers and inflammation

▸ cancer

▸ narrowing, hernia, pouches, or tumors in the esophagus

▸ blockages

▸ growths and scar tissue

Before the test. These tests also call for digestive organs to be empty. To prepare for a barium swallow, you usually avoid eating or drinking anything after midnight the night before the test.

What to expect. You will drink barium, which might remind you of a thick milkshake, just before the X-rays begin. It. As the barium travels through your digestive system, X-rays are taken. The radiologist uses a special X-ray machine called a fluoroscope to view your digestive system. This helps her determine whether it is in good working order.

Word to the wise

A variation of this test is the enteroclysis or small bowel enema. In this test, barium is pumped through a small, flexible tube passed through your nose or mouth and stomach into the beginning of your small intestine. This places the barium directly into the small intestine and may help the doctor spot tumors or signs of diverticular disease or Crohn's disease.

The fluoroscope streams X-rays through your body and projects them onto a fluorescent viewing screen for real-time moving images. As the barium moves into the small intestine, the radiologist can take X-rays of it as well, but this adds more time to the test. A barium swallow takes one to two hours, but X-rays of the small intestine may take three to five hours.

Side effects and risks. You may get more exposure to radiation than from normal X-rays. Also, the barium could build up enough to block your intestines if your body doesn't get rid of it within a day or two. Some people have an allergic reaction to the barium.

After the test. The barium may cause constipation and gray or white stool for a few days. You may be given a laxative to help clear the barium out of your body.

Advantages and disadvantages. The barium swallow gives your doctor more detail than X-rays can, yet it's cheaper than endoscopy. The barium swallow may miss up to 35 percent of ulcers in the small intestine. On a cost scale of 1 to 7 where 7 is the most expensive, this test rates a 3.

Esophageal manometry

The muscles in your esophagus contract to form waves that sweep food down into your stomach, like ocean waves sweep into shore. These waves can be measured and timed by esophageal manometry.

Contractions that are too strong may lead to pain, difficulty swallowing, or even spasms. When contractions are too weak, the bottom end of the esophagus may not close effectively, allowing stomach acid to slip into the esophagus and lead to gastroesophageal reflux.

The test also measures the pressure of the lower esophageal sphincter or LES, the valve at the bottom of the esophagus that keeps stomach acid in your stomach. When LES pressure is too low, stomach acid reflux kicks in. When too high, food may not easily pass into the stomach

Why be tested. Esophageal manometry may be used to diagnose or rule out the following problems:

▶ gastroesophageal reflux

▶ esophageal spasm

▶ achalasia — when the LES can't open to let food into the stomach

Before the test. Tell your doctor about any heartburn medicine or other drugs you regularly take. Avoid alcohol and tobacco for 24 hours before the test. Don't eat or drink anything for at least eight hours before the test.

What to expect. Before the test, someone will take your blood pressure and pulse and spray your throat with a local anesthetic. The technician takes a manometry probe, a long, thin, soft tube that can measure pressure, and threads it through your nose or mouth. Then she guides the probe through your esophagus into your stomach. You may start to gag, but that feeling usually passes quickly.

Word to the wise

This test is necessary if you want to have surgery to correct swallowing difficulties or severe reflux.

While you lie on your side, the technician takes a reading of the pressure in your stomach. Then she slowly withdraws the probe until it reaches the lower part of the esophagus. From time to time, the technician will ask you to swallow a sip of water. Then she'll withdraw the probe until it's in the upper esophagus. After more sips of water, the probe will finally be removed. If you have chest pain, but heart disease has been ruled out, you may be asked to do things that will trigger the pain so the technician can try to find out what's causing it.

Side effects and risks. Inserting the probe through the nose can lead to bleeding, but the risk is minor. The tube may cause you to salivate more. This raises the chance that saliva will accidentally be inhaled into your lungs, which can lead to lung injury or aspiration pneumonia. This is more likely to happen to people who have difficulty swallowing. Stomach contents may also be inadvertently inhaled into the lungs during this test.

After the test. You can return to your normal diet, medications, and activities, but you may have a sore throat.

Advantages and disadvantages. This test is unpleasant and has a high rate of false negatives. On a cost scale of 1 to 7 where 7 is the most expensive, this test rates a 4.

pH testing

These tests detect stomach acid that has sneaked into the esophagus. When it's functioning properly, the lower esophageal sphincter (LES) keeps stomach acid in the stomach.

Why be tested. This test can diagnose or rule out GERD or acid reflux.

Before the test. Tell your doctor about any drugs you take because they can interfere with the test. Avoid alcohol and tobacco for 24 hours before, and don't eat or drink anything for eight hours before.

What to expect. The Bernstein test, or acid perfusion test, is done in the doctor's office. The technician guides the probe through your nose and into your esophagus. Small amounts of salt water and hydrochloric acid are passed through the probe. If the acid seems to trigger chest pain or heartburn but not the salt water, your esophagus may be inflamed. If both cause pain, your esophagus may be too sensitive. If neither hurts, your symptoms probably aren't caused by GERD.

For a more extensive test, the tube of the probe can be attached to a small data recorder that you can carry in a pocket or wear on your wrist. The technician guides the probe through your nose and into your esophagus. As pH measurements are taken, the data recorder saves them. You'll probably be asked to record any symptoms you have during that time. When you return the next day, the data are entered into a computer for analysis. The times when acidity was detected are checked to see if they match your symptoms.

Side effects and risks. The probe insertion carries a slight risk of bleeding.

After the test. You are free to return to your normal diet, medications, and activities.

Advantages and disadvantages. This test is time-consuming and uncomfortable. It can also have a high rate of false negatives. But if other tests have failed to find your problem, this test may help. On a scale of 1 to 7 where 7 is the most expensive, this test rates a 5.

Upper GI endoscopy

Upper GI endoscopy shows the doctor the inside of your esophagus, stomach, and the first part of your small intestine called the duodenum.

This test can help him find out what's causing symptoms like persistent nausea or vomiting, trouble swallowing, loss of appetite, or bloody stools.

Why be tested. Upper GI endoscopy may be used to help diagnose or rule out problems like these:

- cancer of the esophagus or stomach
- peptic ulcer or gastritis caused by *H. pylori*
- malabsorption syndrome — when your small intestine can't adequately absorb nutrients
- bleeding ulcers
- reflux

- inflammation
- Barrett's esophagus

Before the test. Take these steps before your upper endoscopy appointment.

- Tell your doctor which medicines you take, and ask which ones you can take during the hours before the test.

- Make sure you mention any allergies.

- Let him know if you have health problems, such as high blood pressure or conditions of the heart, lung, kidneys, or liver.

- Arrange for someone to take you home after the test.

Your stomach must be empty for the test to be effective and safe. That's why your doctor may tell you not to eat or drink anything for at least six hours before the test. Also avoid antacids, aspirin, or ibuprofen. Advil, Aleve, and Motrin all contain ibuprofen.

What to expect. Right before the test, you'll switch to a hospital gown and remove any eyeglasses, contacts, or dentures. Then the doctor will numb your throat to help reduce gagging. He may also give you pain medicine and a sedative.

The test begins when you swallow the endoscope, a thin, flexible, lighted tube with a camera on the end. Although you may feel like gagging when the test begins, that feeling will pass quickly, and the endoscope won't interfere with breathing. You may also feel some pressure in your abdomen.

The endoscope transmits the camera's images so they can be viewed on a TV screen. The scope may also blow air into your stomach to make it easier to see. Your doctor carefully examines the lining of your

Word to the wise

A key drawback of upper GI endoscopy is that it can't examine the entire small intestine. But a new test called capsule endoscopy can do that without the endoscope.

esophagus, stomach, and duodenum. The scope helps him see problems, like inflammation or bleeding, that don't show up well on X-rays. He can also insert instruments into the endoscope to remove tissue samples, called a biopsy, for testing. In some cases, he may do through-the-scope treatments, like stopping a bleeding problem.

Side effects and risks. Possible complications of upper endoscopy include bleeding, infection, reactions to medication, and perforating or puncturing the stomach lining, esophagus, or small intestine wall, but these are rare. Bleeding and perforations are more likely if a biopsy is part of your test. After the test, your gag reflex may be temporarily repressed so it won't be safe to eat or drink for several hours.

After the test. The test takes 20 to 30 minutes. You must wait up to two hours for the sedative to wear off before you can leave. You may also have to wait several hours to eat or drink — until your gag reflex returns. Most people will have a mild sore throat after the test. Call your doctor immediately if you experience severe stomach pain, fever, increased blood in stools or vomit, extreme dizziness, and difficulty swallowing.

Advantages and disadvantages. Although this test means you can get a biopsy without facing surgery, swallowing the endoscope can be uncomfortable. So can having air pumped into your stomach, if that is part of the test ordered for you. On a 1 to 7 scale where 7 is the most expensive, the cost of this test is a 4.

Capsule endoscopy

This test can examine the entire small intestine without an endoscope. Capsule endoscopy uses a camera in a capsule to transmit images to a recorder.

Why be tested. A capsule endoscopy may be used to diagnose or rule out the following problems:

- Crohn's disease

- polyps

- ulcers

- bleeding

- tumors in the small intestine

- Barrett's esophagus

- severe acid reflux

Before the test. Check with your insurance company to find out whether your policy covers this test.

Avoid all water, other drinks, and all food for 12 hours before the test. Follow your doctor's instructions, and tell him about any medications you take, including iron supplements, aspirin, and other over-the-counter medicines. Also, mention any allergies to medications and medical conditions, such as difficulty swallowing and heart or lung disease. Tell your doctor if you have a pacemaker, inflammatory bowel disease, or if you've had abdominal surgery or a history of blockages in your bowel.

What to expect. According to the American Society for Gastrointestinal Endoscopy, your doctor will apply a sensor device to your abdominal area. Next, you'll swallow the capsule endoscope just like a pill. A data recorder, which you'll wear on your belt for the next eight hours, sends pictures to the recorder while the pill camera passes through your digestive tract.

Unless your doctor has told you otherwise, you can drink clear liquids starting two hours after swallowing the camera, and eat a light meal two hours after that. But avoid strenuous or heavy activities, like running, until the test is over. Be careful not to prematurely disconnect the recorder or pictures will be lost.

Eight hours after you swallowed the camera, you go back to the doctor to have the data recorder removed. Call your doctor immediately if you have unusual bloating, pain, or vomiting during the test.

Side effects and risks. Complications are rare when trained, experienced doctors handle the test. Potential risks include problems with the pill blocking some part of the digestive tract. This can occur if your intestine has been narrowed by inflammation, a tumor, or past surgery.

After the test. Most people go right back to their normal lives after returning the recorder. But tell your doctor immediately if you develop a fever or increasing chest pain after the test or if you have trouble swallowing.

Advantages and disadvantages. This test can cost anywhere from $500 to $2,000 and may not be covered by insurance.

HIDA scan

A HIDA scan can find tiny gallstones or other problems that previous tests have missed. A HIDA scan examines your liver, gallbladder, and bile ducts using X-ray-like pictures. It can even check whether your gallbladder is working properly.

Why be tested. The HIDA scan may be used to help diagnose or rule out problems like these:

- gallbladder infection
- bile duct blockage
- gallstones
- defects of the gallbladder
- tumors or cancer
- cholecystitis (inflammation of the gallbladder)
- bile leaks

Before the test. Be sure to tell your doctor about medications you take. Some drugs can interfere with the test. Also, tell him if you might be pregnant or are breast-feeding. You may be asked to avoid drinking or eating anything for up to eight hours before the test, so plan accordingly.

What to expect. A small amount of radioactive dye will be injected into your arm just before the test begins. You may feel a little pain after the injection, but the rest of the HIDA scan is easy. You just lie beneath a special camera called a scintillation camera or gamma camera. Your natural digestive processes and the camera do all the work. Your liver pulls the dye from your bloodstream and passes it through your gallbladder and bile ducts while the camera catches it all on film. A computer processes and stores the images. The test normally takes one to two hours.

Side effects and risks. The risks and side effects from a HIDA scan are temporary and minor. Some people have a reaction to the radioactive dye, but that's rare. The amount of radioactivity you're exposed to is very small and leaves your system quickly.

After the test. Your arm may be a little sore from the injection, but you can go back to your normal activities.

Advantages and disadvantages. The HIDA scan is very good at uncovering gallbladder inflammation and poor gallbladder contraction. However, it often detects problems, but not the cause. What's more, false positives can be a problem. That means it probably won't be the only test you need. High amounts of bilirubin in your blood may affect the results. On a scale of 1 to 7 where 7 is the most expensive, this test rates a 5.

ERCP

Endoscopic retrograde cholangiopancreatography or ERCP is a valuable tool. It's used to examine the stomach and duodenum, the upper part of the small intestine.

Why be tested. Doctors often use it to find, or rule out, these problems:

- blockage or narrowing of the bile ducts
- pancreatitis
- blockage or narrowing of the pancreatic duct
- cancer

ERCP may also help diagnose and treat other problems in the liver, bile duct, gallbladder, and pancreas.

Before the test. Make sure you give this information to your doctor before having an ERCP.

- a list of your allergies, including drug allergies or reactions, especially to iodine, which is in the contrast dye
- names of all medications you take, including blood thinners and aspirin-containing drugs
- any health problems, in particular heart or lung conditions

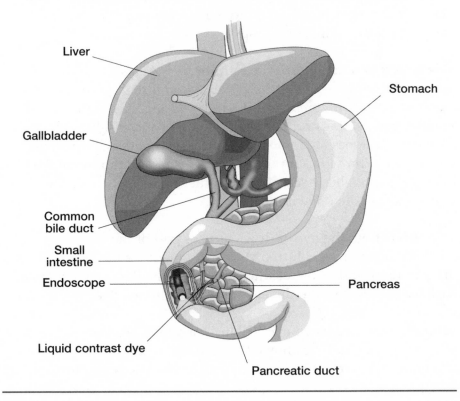

Liver

Stomach

Gallbladder

Common bile duct

Small intestine

Endoscope

Pancreas

Liquid contrast dye

Pancreatic duct

To prepare for the ERCP, you'll be instructed not to eat anything for eight hours prior to the test. Before starting the procedure, your doctor will give you a sedative. He might also provide painkillers and medicine to numb the back of your throat. Remember to arrange for someone to drive you home. Because of the sedative, you won't be allowed to drive.

What to expect. The ERCP starts when you swallow an endoscope — a thin, flexible tube tipped with a tiny camera and light. The camera transmits images to a nearby television monitor. Your doctor guides the scope through your esophagus. Then he examines the lining of your stomach and duodenum.

Your doctor inserts a tiny tube through the endoscope. When it reaches the point where the bile ducts and pancreatic duct open into the duodenum, he directs the scope into the appropriate duct. After sending a liquid contrast dye through to the duct to make it more visible, he examines and photographs the duct with X-ray equipment. This helps pinpoint widening, narrowing, or blockage of the duct. The endoscope can also be used to remove gallstones or scar tissue and take a tissue sample for biopsy.

Side effects and risks. ERCP takes from 30 minutes to two hours. You may experience some fullness or discomfort, but the endoscope won't interfere with breathing. The most common complication of ERCP is pancreatitis or inflammation of the pancreas. Bleeding can also occur if stones are removed, scar tissue is cut away, or stents — tubes used to provide support — are inserted. Perforation of the bile duct is also possible if scar tissue or other tissue is cut away to widen the bile duct opening.

Side effects from the dye or drugs used as part of the test may include nausea, hives, blurred vision, dry mouth, a burning or flushing sensation, and urine retention. People with allergies to iodine or shellfish may have a life-threatening reaction to the dye.

After the test. Unless your ERCP includes gallstone removal or other surgery, you'll be allowed to go home in an hour or two, when the sedative wears off. Your doctor will check you for signs of complications before you leave. Expect temporary aftereffects, such as feeling full, passing gas, soft stools, or changes in bowel habits. Call your doctor if you notice bleeding from your rectum, fever over 100 degrees, vomiting, severe abdominal pain, weakness, dizziness, or black, tarry stools.

Advantages and disadvantages. Some problems ERCP finds can also be treated through the endoscope. For example, a stone blocking one of the ducts can often be removed. Also, tissue samples can be taken for testing. If gallstones are removed by the endoscope, you may be able to avoid surgery. ERCP is considered safer than percutaneous transhepatic cholangiography (PTHC). Although ERCP has been considered the best choice for images of bile ducts, MRCP may also be used, and it might have fewer risks. On a scale of 1 to 7 where 7 is the most expensive, this test rates a 4.

Magnetic resonance cholangiopancreatography (MRCP)

MRCP helps doctors examine the bile duct, the pancreatic duct, and the gallbladder. Magnetic resonance imaging (MRI) technology helps make this possible. A large, tube-shaped MRI machine forms a strong magnetic field around you. The field combines with a radio frequency and computers to create images. It can even make cross-section pictures for more detail. In fact, MRCP is accurate enough to sometimes replace endoscopic retrograde cholangiopancreatography (ERCP) — a test that requires you to swallow a long, thin tube called an endoscope.

Why be tested. Conditions that affect the bile ducts, gallbladder, pancreas, and pancreatic duct are an MRCP specialty. This test may be used to diagnose or rule out problems like these:

▸ gallstones

▸ pancreatitis caused by gallstones

▸ tumors or cancer

▸ defects in the bile ducts or pancreatic ducts

▸ inflammation and narrowing of bile ducts

▸ complications of chronic pancreatitis, such as a narrowed duct

Before the test. Be sure to tell your doctor or the MRCP technician if you have a pacemaker, inner ear implants, brain aneurysm clips, artificial heart valves, vascular stents, artificial joints, insulin pumps, shrapnel, or any other metal in your body. The MRCP is not safe for some people because its strong magnetic field can disturb or interrupt the actions of implanted metal objects or devices.

Don't take eyeglasses, removable dental work, or other metal objects into the MRI room. Credit cards, hearing aids, jewelry, and watches can be damaged by the magnets. Metal in items like hairpins and zippers can distort MRCP images.

Do not eat or drink anything for at least four hours before the test. A full stomach can interfere with the pictures of your bile or pancreatic ducts.

Some people struggle with claustrophobia while inside the MRI scanner. If you're one of them, ask for a sedative. You can also ask about earplugs if the noise of the machine bothers you.

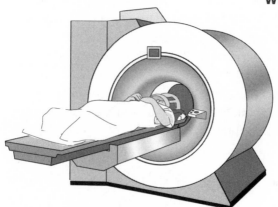

What to expect. An MRI technician will take you to the MRI table to begin the scan. She'll put a coil around your waist like a belt. This will act like an antenna to make the images more clear during the scan. The MRI staff won't stay in the

room with you, but they'll be able to see and hear you. And you'll be able to hear their instructions.

Side effects and risks. Although MRIs don't have side effects or complications, they're not recommended for pregnant women or anyone who has metal implants or other metal in the body.

After the test. MRCP takes about 10 minutes, and you shouldn't experience any aftereffects from the test.

Advantages and disadvantages. MRCP is less invasive than ERCP but may not be as widely available. Gallstone removal, biopsies, and removal of scar tissue cannot be done with MRCP. In addition, since other MRI tests average between $700 and $1,000, the MRCP could be expensive. On the other hand, MRCP produces images that are almost as good as ERCP, but without the risk of pancreatitis, problems from sedation, or tears in digestive organs. MRCP can serve as a replacement for ERCP when the risks of using ERCP are high or when treatment via an endoscope would not be useful.

Ultrasound

You don't have to be pregnant to get important news from an ultrasound. It's also used to check the kidneys, liver, gallbladder, pancreas, spleen, and blood vessels of the abdomen. Ultrasound creates pictures of internal organs by gently bouncing high-frequency sound waves off the organs your doctor needs to see. The reflected sound waves' echoes are recorded and displayed as a picture.

The images are captured in real time so they can show internal movement, like blood flow. This can help diagnose a variety of conditions and problems.

Why be tested. An abdominal ultrasound may be used to diagnose or rule out many problems like these:

- gallstones

- kidney stones

- cholecystitis (gallbladder inflammation)

- pancreatitis

- inflamed appendix

- tumors

- fluid build-up in the abdomen

Before the test. Your doctor may tell you not to eat or drink for up to 12 hours before the test. For a gallbladder scan, the meal before the 12-hour fast begins must be fat free.

What to expect. An ultrasound is quick, simple, and pain free. You will lie on your back on an examining table or reclining chair. The sonographer will spread water-based lubricating gel across your abdomen to help transmit sound waves.

Then, she'll press a small, hand-held device, called a transducer, firmly against your abdomen, moving it until the images are captured. You may be asked to hold your breath for short periods of time during the test. As the sonographer guides the transducer over your abdominal area, you may have some discomfort from the pressure, especially if you have a full bladder.

Throughout the exam, every ultrasound image is immediately visible on a nearby screen. The sonographer watches this screen to help her do her job, but you can usually see it as well.

Side effects and risks. Unlike tests with radiation or X-rays, ultrasound is not risky.

After the test. Ultrasound has no aftereffects so you can get right back to normal as soon as the test is done.

Advantages and disadvantages. The ultrasound is probably the most sensitive test for finding gallstones. This test is radiation free and less expensive than a CT scan, but it doesn't produce as clear a picture. Intestinal gas can block the ultrasound's view of the pancreas and bile ducts. People who are obese may also end up with lower-quality images. Extra tissue weakens the sound waves as they pass into the body. On a scale of 1 to 7 where 7 is the most expensive, ultrasound rates a 3.

Word to the wise

A new kind of test called endoscopic ultrasound combines ultrasound with endoscopy. A tiny ultrasound probe is attached to a tube called an endoscope. The endoscope is inserted into the digestive tract. The ultrasound probe can be swept over the organ that needs to be examined. For example, the pancreas can be harder to view clearly with regular ultrasound because the bowel gets in the way. And tissues or gas are far less likely to dim the view with endoscopic ultrasound.

PTHC

This test helps determine what may be blocking the bile duct system. After being lightly sedated, you lie on an X-ray table while a needle is inserted through your skin and liver and into your bile duct. Dye injected through the needle helps the bile duct system show up on X-rays. Although this is somewhat uncomfortable, the blockage can be drained during this test so you may avoid surgery.

Complications include allergic reaction to the dye, bleeding, infection, and a possible bile leak into the abdominal cavity. On a scale of 1 to 7 where 7 is the most expensive, this test rates a 5.

Fecal occult blood test (FOBT)

The FOBT is an easy, painless stool test that detects small amounts of hidden blood in your stool. The FOBT is best known for colon cancer screening because blood can be a sign of cancer or cancerous growths called polyps. FOBT also checks for bleeding from the entire digestive tract.

Why be tested. The FOBT may be used to diagnose or rule out the following problems:

- ulcers
- polyps or cancer
- inflammatory bowel disease
- hemorrhoids
- gastritis
- dilated or twisted veins

Before the test. Tell your doctor about all prescription and over-the-counter drugs and supplements you take. You might need to stop taking some of them a few days before the test.

For more accurate results, your doctor may ask you to follow these instructions starting three days before the test and continuing through the testing period.

- *Don't eat* red meat.
- *Avoid bananas, cantaloupes, apples,* oranges, and grapes, cauliflower, turnips, horseradish, artichokes, mushrooms, radishes, broccoli, and bean sprouts.

> *Don't take vitamin C supplements* or eat large amounts of citrus fruits.

> *Eat high-fiber foods,* like whole grains and vegetables, to increase the bulk of stools.

> *Avoid iron supplements,* antacids, steroids, and nonsteroidal anti-inflammatory drugs (NSAIDs), like aspirin and ibuprofen.

> *Avoid alcohol and anything* else that can irritate your bowels and stomach.

> *Consider this.* If your gums usually bleed when you brush your teeth, try not to brush for three days before the test.

What to expect. This is an at-home test. You'll be given a test kit to take home and specific instructions on how to use it for the most accurate results. Usually, you are responsible for collecting the stool samples for several days, possibly in a clear plastic container. You may also be asked to use a special stick to dab a little of the sample on a special card. These samples will be analyzed by a laboratory.

Side effects and risks. This test is free of side effects and risks.

After the test. You can go back to normal activities. The diet and drug restrictions usually end when the test does.

Advantages and disadvantages. This test is painless and easy, but false positives and false negatives are common. Only 60 percent of colon cancers are found with this test. That means you could miss the chance to catch polyps or cancer early. Collecting samples is unpleasant, and the test cannot give you a specific and definite diagnosis. Testing positive means more tests. On a scale of 1 to 7, this test rates a 3.

Word to the wise

Make sure you eat extra fiber before the test. It helps make tumors or polyps bleed if they're present. If you're tempted to eat meat, remember it can contain blood, which may cause a false reading.

Sigmoidoscopy

A flexible sigmoidoscopy is an accurate way for your doctor to inspect your rectum and the lower part of your colon, called the sigmoid or descending colon. The instrument he uses is called a sigmoidoscope, a short, flexible, lighted tube with a camera at the end.

Why be tested. Sigmoidoscopy can be used to diagnose or rule out problems like these:

- polyps and other abnormal growths
- colon cancer
- bleeding
- fissures or hemorrhoids
- inflammation
- intestinal ulcers
- diverticular disease

Before the test. The colon and rectum must be completely empty for flexible sigmoidoscopy to be effective and safe. Follow your doctor's instructions carefully about what foods to avoid before the test. He may also ask you to take a laxative.

Tell your doctor about any medications you're taking, particularly aspirin-containing drugs or anticoagulants (blood thinners), as well as any drug allergies you have. Also, mention whether you need to take antibiotics before dental procedures.

What to expect. Flexible sigmoidoscopy is usually done without sedatives or painkillers. While you lie on your side on the exam table, the doctor inserts the sigmoidoscope into your rectum and slowly guides it into your colon. The scope blows air into your rectum and colon to inflate them so he can see them better. This can cause pressure, bloating, and cramping.

Your doctor carefully examines the lining of your colon as he gradually withdraws the sigmoidoscope. If he sees anything abnormal, like a small polyp, he can remove it using instruments inserted into the scope and send it to the lab for examination.

Side effects and risks. Complications are rare, but they can include bleeding, infection, and a small risk of colon perforation. In one study, approximately 14 percent of the people who had a sigmoidoscopy experienced pain, 3 percent had bleeding, and 25 percent had gas.

After the test. Flexible sigmoidoscopy takes 10 to 20 minutes. Normal aftereffects include bloating or mild cramping from the air passed into the colon during the test. This will vanish quickly when you pass gas. But if you notice severe abdominal pain, fevers and chills, or rectal bleeding of more than one-half cup, contact your doctor immediately.

Advantages and disadvantages. Flexible sigmoidoscopy allows your doctor to examine your rectum and sigmoid or descending colon. This test is usually done without sedatives or painkillers. While it's cheaper and faster than a colonoscopy, the sigmoidoscope can't examine the entire colon. This means it can't find cancer or polyps in the upper colon, unlike a colonoscopy. This is particularly important if you have a family history of colon cancer or other risk factors.

If a polyp is found during sigmoidoscopy, your doctor might recommend a colonoscopy. Some polyps can lead to cancer. The colonoscopy can remove large polyps and check the rest of your colon. On a scale of 1 to 7 where 7 is the most expensive, this test rates a 3.

Colonoscopy

Just one colonoscopy may reduce your colon cancer risk up to 60 percent over the next 10 years if you're over 50, according to a study from researchers at the University of California, San Francisco, and the University of Michigan Health System. However, although colonoscopy is the most accurate and useful test for spotting colon

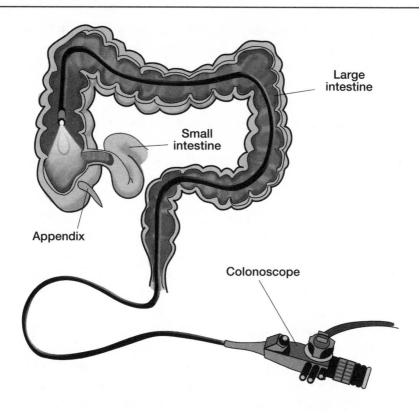

cancer and polyps that may be precancerous, it requires sedation. Some medical authorities doubt that the benefits outweigh the risks in screening people who are symptom-free. A colonoscopy can also uncover the cause of mysterious changes in bowel habits, which may be symptoms of other problems.

Why be tested. A colonoscopy can help diagnose or rule out the following problems:

- inflammatory bowel disease
- intestinal ulcers
- diverticulosis
- bleeding in the intestine
- polyps or other abnormal growths
- colitis
- colon cancer

Before the test. The better you prepare for a colonoscopy, the more accurate it will be. Tell your doctor about any health problems you have, including allergies, and any medications and supplements you take. People who have had a recent heart attack or abdominal surgery cannot safely undergo colonoscopy. You also need to avoid colonoscopy if you've had a tear in your bowel or if you have diverticulitis.

Carefully follow all instructions your doctor gives you, especially about cleaning out your colon. This may involve a special diet, laxatives, or enemas, so plan your activities accordingly. Also, because you will be sedated, arrange for someone to take you home after the test.

What to expect. After giving you a painkiller and a sedative, the doctor will perform a quick rectal exam before inserting a colonoscope into your rectum. The colonoscope is a lighted, flexible tube equipped with a camera. Your doctor can direct the camera view, which displays on a TV monitor. If he finds abnormalities in your colon, he can also take a biopsy, remove a suspicious growth, or stop bleeding through the colonoscope.

Side effects and risks. Side effects of colonoscopy may include gas, cramps, and feeling the urge for a bowel movement. Complications are rare but may include heavy bleeding from biopsy or growth removal or perforation of the colon wall. Bleeding occurs in up to 25 cases out of every 1,000 colonoscopy exams. Perforations occur in up to 4 out of every 1,000 colonoscopies that require no polyp removal or other surgery.

Word to the wise

Medicare covers colonoscopy — for people who are eligible — once every 10 years for those over 50 who aren't at high risk, or once every two years for a person of any age who's at high risk. You're at high risk if you or an immediate family member has had colon cancer or a suspicious polyp. Anyone with inflammatory bowel disease is also high risk. Medicare also covers a colonoscopy needed to confirm or deny possible cancer or polyps found by another test.

Perforations occur in up to 10 out of every 1,000 polyp removals during colonoscopy.

After the test. Most colonoscopies take an hour or less, but plan to spend an hour or two recovering from the sedative. After that, you can ask your doctor about the test results and get directions for returning to a normal diet. By 24 hours after your colonoscopy, minor symptoms, like bloating, gas, or mild cramping, should vanish. Contact your doctor if you notice severe abdominal pain, fever, chills, or more than a half cup of rectal bleeding.

Advantages and disadvantages. The person who gives you a colonoscopy must be more highly trained than people responsible for other kinds of colon cancer screening. But some experts worry that the current number of colonoscopy technicians won't be enough if demand for colonoscopies increases. On a scale of 1 to 7 where 7 is the most expensive, this test rates a 4.

A recent study found that people who drank a portion of a polyethylene glycol (PEG) bowel-cleansing solution every 10 minutes, followed by five minutes of walking — until they finished the recommended amount of the solution — were more likely to have a well-cleansed colon. This is very important for accurate and valid test results. The procedure worked best for younger adults who were not obese.

Preparing the bowel can be very unpleasant. For these reasons and more, a report from the Agency for Healthcare Research and Quality (AHRQ) states it's hard to tell whether colonoscopy is right for everyone. Yet, colonoscopy covers more of the colon than a sigmoidoscopy, and the sedative and painkiller can make the colonoscopy more comfortable for you.

According to the U.S. Preventive Services Task Force, scientists aren't sure how accurate colonoscopy is. Estimates suggest colonoscopy finds 90 percent of large polyps and 75 percent of small ones. But the Task Force report also says that only a

Compare colon cancer screening choices

Advantages	Disadvantages
Fecal occult blood test (FOBT)	
• Noninvasive • Low cost	• False-positive and false negative results are common. • The test is unpleasant. • If you test positive, you'll need more tests.
Sigmoidoscopy	
• Easy • Inexpensive • Highly accurate in examining the lower third of the colon.	• Only one-third or less of the colon is examined, so cancers in the rest of colon may be missed. • It's usually done without sedatives or painkillers. • You may still need a colonoscopy if any problems are found. • Rare complications, like intestinal perforation or bleeding, are possible.
Colonoscopy	
• Most reliable • Examines entire colon • Can remove abnormal growths and polyps during the exam	• It's expensive. • Rare complications, like intestinal perforation or bleeding, are possible. • This test should be avoided if you've had a recent heart attack or abdominal surgery. • The preparation and procedure is uncomfortable for most people. • A poorly cleansed bowel can affect test results. • It should not be done if bowel tears are suspected or in cases of acute diverticulitis. • There's a small risk of infection.

Continued

Compare colon cancer screening choices

Advantages	Disadvantages
Double-contrast barium enema (DCBE)	
• Less expensive • Examines entire colon • Detailed picture with double-contrast barium enema • Under some conditions, can be substituted for flexible sigmoidoscopy or colonoscopy	• It won't detect as many large polyps or early cancers as colonoscopy. • Smaller cancers and precancerous areas may be missed. • A colonoscopy must be done to take a biopsy, remove a growth, or confirm any polyp, tumor, or other problem found by a barium enema. • It's less expensive, painful, and invasive than colonoscopy. • There's a small risk of bowel tear. • You may experience discomfort during or after the exam. • Barium can cause extreme constipation.
Virtual colonoscopy	
• Takes less time than a regular colonoscopy or barium enema. • May be more comfortable for some people • No sedatives	• Medicare does not reimburse virtual colonoscopy costs for colon cancer screening. • The doctor can't take tissue samples, remove polyps, or do any other treatment, so you may need to have a colonoscopy, too. • It may show less detail than regular colonoscopy, so some polyps may not be detected • You're given no sedatives or painkillers, but having air pumped into your colon can be painful. • No one is sure how often VC should be done to lower cancer risk. Researchers also don't know whether doing VC as often as regular colonoscopy would carry radiation risks.

minority of the polyps detected or removed during colonoscopy would have developed into cancer.

On the other hand, colon cancer kills more than 55,000 people each year. Fortunately, the cure rates are high — 90 percent of all cases — when this cancer is caught early.

If you're at average risk for colon cancer, the American Cancer Society (ACS) recommends beginning screening at age 50 with one or more of these methods:

▶ fecal occult blood test (FOBT) annually. (However, new research suggests this is a poor screening method when used alone.)

▶ flexible sigmoidoscopy every five years.

▶ annual FOBT plus flexible sigmoidoscopy every five years.

▶ double-contrast barium enema every five years.

▶ colonoscopy every 10 years.

But not everyone agrees with the ACS recommendation that everyone over 50 should have a colonoscopy. Nortin M. Hadler, M.D., medical school professor and author of the book *The Last Well Person*, points out that colon cancer spreads more slowly than some other cancers. At age 50, he says, you have about a 2-percent chance of dying from colon cancer over the next 30 years, compared to a 60-percent chance of dying from anything else during those years. Hadler has had a less-risky sigmoidoscopy that examines the lower part of the colon that is most at risk for cancer. He chooses to avoid the risks of the more thorough colonoscopy that most gastroenterologists recommend. Yet, he believes each person must make his own decision about colonoscopy.

Barium enema

These tests use X-rays to examine your digestive tract for diseases, conditions, and malfunctions. A lower GI series checks for trouble in your colon and rectum. The test requires barium — a liquid that helps organs show up more clearly on X-rays. If the barium enema is a double-contrast barium enema (DCBE), air is added to the colon to help the barium coat the colon wall. This makes it easier for the radiologist to see small tumors and polyps.

Why be tested. The lower GI series may be used to diagnose or rule out problems like these:

- Crohn's disease
- diverticular disease
- bleeding in the intestines
- polyps and tumors
- inflammatory bowel disease
- intestinal ulcers

Before the test. You might be limited to liquids and nondairy foods for two days before the test and clear liquids the day before. As with the upper GI series, you avoid food and drink after midnight the night before. To make sure your colon is empty, you may be given a laxative or an enema before the test.

What to expect. The radiologist will put barium into your colon before taking X-rays. The barium will cause fullness, pressure, and the urge to have a bowel movement, but the urge will pass. You'll be able to go to the bathroom after the X-rays, but the radiologist may want X-rays of the empty colon afterward. Plan for the lower GI series to take up to two hours.

Side effects and risks. A survey suggests that serious complications only occur in 1 in 10,000 examinations. The survey also found that bowel perforations occurred in 1 in 25,000 barium enemas and death in 1 out of 55,000 tests.

After the test. The barium may cause constipation and gray or white stool for a few days.

Advantages and disadvantages. Although the double-contrast barium enema (DCBE) can be used for colon cancer screening, studies suggest that the accuracy rate of this test may range from 48 percent to 90 percent. The DCBE won't detect as many large polyps or early cancers as colonoscopy, and it could miss smaller cancers and precancerous areas. A colonoscopy might be needed to obtain a biopsy or remove an abnormal growth found by a barium enema.

Other disadvantages include the same uncomfortable bowel preparation as for colonoscopy, possible discomfort during and after the exam, and the ability to cause severe constipation. In addition, you cannot take this test if you have a suspected bowel tear or may have acute diverticulitis.

DCBE is cheaper than colonoscopy, examines the entire colon, and shows the colon wall in good detail. It's also less painful than colonoscopy, less invasive, and may be a reasonable alternative for some people who can't undergo colonoscopy or sigmoidoscopy. On a scale of 1 to 7 where 7 is the most expensive, this test rates a 3.

Virtual colonoscopy

Virtual colonoscopy (VC) combines X-rays and computers to generate images of your entire colon. VC can be done with computed tomography (CT) or with magnetic resonance imaging (MRI).

Why be tested. Virtual colonoscopy helps doctors diagnose or rule out problems like these:

- ▶ polyps
- ▶ diverticular disease
- ▶ colon cancer

Before the test. Your colon must be empty for VC to be effective, so follow your doctor's instructions carefully. She may ask you to take laxatives and go on a clear liquid diet the day before the test. She

Word to the wise

One study that reported high accuracy in virtual colonoscopy used an advanced CT scanner, special training for radiologists, and other techniques that aren't commonly available with most VCs. VC may compete more effectively with colonoscopy if advantages like these become more widely available. Future technological improvements may also improve the accuracy of VC.

might even prescribe a suppository to help cleanse your colon.

What to expect. In a hospital, you'll lie on a table that's attached to a CT or MRI scanner. A thin tube will be inserted into your rectum, and air will be pumped through it. This inflates your colon and makes it easier to examine fully. The table will glide through the scanner to rapidly create a series of pictures of the entire colon. The technician may ask you to hold your breath to avoid blurring the images. You'll turn to lie on your stomach for a second photo shoot. The test takes about 10 minutes.

Side effects and risks. If the scan is done with a CT scanner, you face the same risks as you would for a normal CT scan.

After the test. Your doctor may ask you to wait for the test results. If you need a regular colonoscopy because problems are found, you may be able to get it the same day and avoid another round of bowel cleansing. You can learn more about this procedure in the *Colonoscopy* section in this chapter.

Advantages and disadvantages. Virtual colonoscopy has these advantages over regular colonoscopy.

▸ VC may be more comfortable for some people because it doesn't require a colonoscope. That also means no sedatives, so you don't need time to recover, and you can drive yourself home.

▸ VC takes less time than a regular colonoscopy or double-contrast barium enema.

VC also has these disadvantages.

▸ At least 30 percent of the people tested with VC need a colonoscopy afterward. That's because a doctor can't take tissue samples, remove polyps, or do any other treatment during VC.

▸ VC may show less detail than regular colonoscopy, so some polyps may not be detected. Although some studies suggest VC can be as accurate as regular colonoscopy, no one is sure.

▸ Medicare does not cover VC, and insurance companies rarely do.

▸ You're given no sedatives or painkillers and having air pumped into your colon can be painful.

▸ No one is sure how often VC should be done to lower cancer risk, but it probably can't be done less often than regular colonoscopy. Researchers also don't know whether doing VC frequently using a CT scanner would carry radiation risks.

▸ According to one study, switching from colonoscopy to VC wouldn't necessarily save lives. For every 100,000 people who switched, three or four would be saved from death due to bowel perforation by the colonoscope, but four or five would die from cancer because VC might not spot the cancer early enough.

Anoscopy

Anoscopy uses an anoscope, a thin plastic tube about 3 inches long, to examine the lower part of the rectum and anus. The anoscopy may be used to diagnose or rule out problems like these:

▸ rectal bleeding

▸ hemorrhoids

▸ tumors

▸ polyps

In some cases, you may be asked to take a laxative or given an enema before the test. The doctor inserts the lubricated anoscope into your anus and rectum. Most people feel pressure, but little or no pain. However, you may feel pain if a problem has made your rectum or anus tender or a biopsy is taken. The exam takes place as the scope is slowly withdrawn.

The anoscope can be used to quickly perform a biopsy or to cauterize an area, if needed. (Cauterizing destroys tissue using electricity, chemicals, heat, or freezing). If the doctor performed a biopsy or cauterization, he will give you specific instructions. Complications are rare but include introducing bacteria into the colon, bleeding, and perforation of the colon or rectal wall. On a scale of 1 to 7 where 7 is the most expensive, this test rates a 1.

Anorectal manometry

This test examines the muscles that control your bowel movements. A probe inserted into your anal canal measures the pressure exerted by those muscles. Pressure that's too high may cause constipation, while pressure that is too low can lead to fecal incontinence. This test can help locate problems in the functioning of the rectal muscles or nerves.

Why be tested. Anorectal manometry may be used to diagnose or rule out the following problems:

- ▸ the cause of chronic constipation or fecal incontinence
- ▸ Hirschsprung's disease, in which chronic constipation is caused by a defect in the nerves that control the colon

Anorectal manometry is not necessary for most people with fecal incontinence. Your doctor probably won't order this test unless he suspects muscle or nerve damage from Hirschsprung's disease, surgery, or a systemic disease, like diabetes or scleroderma.

Before the test. Tell your doctor if you have an allergy to latex or rubber. You can't take this test if you do. You may be given an enema to clear any feces from the rectum. If you are very anxious before the test, your doctor may give you a sedative.

What to expect. You lie on an examining table and the doctor does a quick rectal exam with a gloved finger. The actual test can be done with one of two instruments.

▸ The regular manometry probe is a thin tube with an instrument that measures pressure. The doctor inserts the probe into your rectum and slowly withdraws it as it measures the pressure exerted by your anal and rectal muscles.

▸ The balloon manometry system is a hollow metal cylinder with three balloons attached. The doctor asks you to squeeze your anus as hard as you can, while pressure is recorded. Next, the doctor inflates a balloon at the tip of the probe, and asks if you feel the urge to have a bowel movement.

Side effects and risks. Some people may be at risk for an allergic reaction to the latex manometry balloon.

After the test. You are free to return to your regular activities.

Advantages and disadvantages. The test is uncomfortable, but it might be a way to avoid a biopsy of muscle tissue. On a scale of 1 to 7 where 7 is the most expensive, this test rates a 2.

Word to the wise

Anorectal manometry is also used to help stop fecal incontinence. It can be used to retrain anal muscles to contract more forcefully.

Transit studies

Transit studies can determine how well food moves through your digestive system. It may be used to find a cause for unexplained weight loss, abdominal pain, bloating, vomiting, nausea, diarrhea, or constipation. It may also detect a blockage in your digestive tract. This test is also used to rule out gastroparesis, which means your stomach empties too slowly. You are at high risk for gastroparesis if you have diabetes.

After fasting overnight, you go to your doctor's office to eat a breakfast of bread and eggs with a glass of milk. The eggs are mixed with a few drops of a slightly radioactive tracer substance, but you won't be able to see or taste it.

The technician will ask you to stand or lie on your back. Then, special cameras, called gamma radiation cameras, will take pictures of the eggs as they pass through your stomach into your small intestine. The first pictures are taken right after you eat, followed by more pictures after one hour, two hours, and four hours. If small bowel transit is also part of your test, more pictures are taken at six hours.

Each picture session only takes five minutes. Between sessions, you can sit or walk. If your stomach is emptying normally, your stomach should be mostly empty after four hours. If your small intestine is emptying normally, at least half the eggs will have left your small intestine by the sixth hour.

A whole-gut transit study works a little differently because you swallow a capsule that contains a radioactive tracer before you eat the tracer eggs. After that the test is just like the stomach and small bowel transit study except you come back for more pictures the next day. That's when the tracer capsule can be followed through your colon.

Like the HIDA scan, this test exposes you to a small amount of radiation. Complications are rare but may include a bad reaction to the radioactive material.

Paracentesis

Fluid can accumulate in the spaces between your abdominal organs. Called ascites, it's usually a sign that something is wrong. Your doctor can withdraw this fluid using a needle and send it to a lab for analysis.

Why be tested. A paracentesis may be used to diagnose or rule out problems like these:

- liver diseases, including cirrhosis
- pancreatitis
- infection
- cancer
- fungal or parasitic diseases
- congestive heart failure

Paracentesis is also used to remove fluid from the abdomen to relieve pressure on your abdominal organs, which will improve digestion.

Before the test. Tell your doctor if you've ever had extensive abdominal surgery. That usually means you shouldn't have a paracentesis. Also, tell him if you're taking antibiotics or other medicines. Don't consume food or drink for at least 12 hours before the test.

What to expect. After emptying your bladder, you lie on your back on an examining table. An area slightly below the navel may be shaved. The doctor will give you local anesthesia to numb your abdominal area.

After the anesthetic takes effect, the doctor inserts a needle into your abdomen. You may feel pressure or a little pain. The doctor may use a CT scan or abdominal ultrasound to help guide the needle. He aims the needle into the peritoneal space — the area surrounding the intestines and other abdominal organs — to draw a sample of fluids.

If you only have a little fluid, the doctor may ask you to get on your hands and knees so the fluid will move to the front of your abdomen. If you have a lot of fluid, the doctor may switch from a syringe to tubes that can drain the fluid into bottles. The tubes, or the needle, are removed once the test is done.

Side effects and risks. Risks include bleeding, swelling, infection, accidental injury to internal organs or blood vessels with the needle, and a drop in blood pressure if too much fluid is removed too quickly. Use of CT scanning may add risks that typically come with a CT scan. Complications are rare, but they may include hemorrhage and infection.

After the test. A doctor or nurse will put a pressure dressing on the incision site and check for leaking. If fluid is leaking, stay calm and lie on your back until it stops. You'll stay in a recovery area for several hours while your heart, blood pressure, breathing, and temperature are monitored.

Advantages and disadvantages. Paracentesis is a relatively safe way to relieve pressure in the abdominal area, and it isn't as invasive as surgery. Yet, you do run the risk of infection, and it won't give your doctor as much useful information as he could get from a laparoscopy or biopsy. On a scale of 1 to 7 where 7 is the most expensive, this test rates a 3.

Laparoscopy

Laparoscopy uses a rigid, fiber-optic tube called a laparoscope to help the doctor view your abdominal organs. This test can help determine why fluids have built up in your abdominal cavity.

Why be tested. A laparoscopy may be used to diagnose or rule out the following problems:

▶ cancer

- cysts
- abscesses
- inflammation
- adhesions

Before the test. Tell your doctor if you take nonsteroidal anti-inflammatory drugs, like aspirin or ibuprofen, or anticoagulants, like warfarin. Also, tell him about any other prescription or over-the-counter medicines and supplements you take. You might need to stop taking them one to two weeks before the test. Tell your doctor if you've had multiple surgeries in your abdominal area, which can make laparoscopy risky. If the laparoscopy will include general anesthesia, you may have an EKG (electrocardiogram) and a chest X-ray before the test. Arrange for someone to take you home a few hours after the test.

What to expect. You'll empty your bladder before the test begins. The area where the laparoscope will be inserted may be shaved. You lie on your back on a table. Then you're given either general anesthesia or a mild sedative followed by local anesthesia. Most laparoscopies require general anesthesia.

Once you are sedated, the doctor inserts a special needle into your abdominal cavity, just below your navel. She pumps air through the needle so your organs are easier to see. In some cases, carbon dioxide or nitrous oxide may be used instead of air. Then the doctor removes the needle. Next, she inserts the laparoscope.

If you are awake, she may ask you to change positions from time to time so she can see your organs more clearly. She may also insert instruments through the laparoscope to take fluid or tissue samples. After the test is done, the doctor removes the laparoscope, lets all the extra air escape out of your abdominal cavity, and stitches the incision closed.

Side effects and risks. You may experience pain in your abdominal area and right shoulder. Serious complications are rare, but they can include infection, perforation of your internal organs, or rupture of your aorta. If general anesthesia is used, other complications may be possible.

After the test. You'll stay in the recovery area for at least several hours while the medical staff monitors your heart rate, breathing, blood pressure, and temperature. You can usually be taken home once the anesthesia wears off.

Avoid drinking carbonated beverages for about two days. They can interact with the gases added to your abdominal cavity during the test. Call your doctor if you have severe pain, bleeding from the incision, or fever.

Advantages and disadvantages. This test is invasive and uncomfortable. However, it may allow your doctor to take a biopsy without doing major surgery. Laparoscopy usually provides enough information so you won't need more tests. On a scale of 1 to 7 where 7 is the most expensive, this test rates a 5.

Intubation of the digestive tract

Intubation of the digestive tract can be used for testing or as a treatment. The doctor passes a small, flexible plastic tube through your nose or mouth, into your esophagus, and down to your stomach or small intestine.

Intubation can check for blood in your stomach or remove a sample of fluids from your small intestine. It also helps determine the acidity of stomach fluids or the source of food poisoning. Sometimes the tube is left in for several hours so multiple samples of stomach fluid can be taken. Intubation is also used to remove fluid and gas from the stomach or small intestine, to feed people who can't swallow, or to remove poison from the stomach.

Although intubation can cause gagging and nausea for some people, a tube inserted through the nose may cause less irritation and coughing.

Abdominal angiography

This test uses contrast dye to help show your digestive tract's blood vessels and blood flow on moving X-rays.

Why be tested. The abdominal angiography may be used to diagnose or rule out the following problems:

- blood vessel disease in the intestines
- a narrowed or blocked artery
- blood vessel abnormalities in the liver or spleen
- cancer
- internal bleeding
- aneurysm in the digestive tract

Before the test. Tell your doctor if you have any allergies, especially if you're allergic to seafood or iodine. You could have a harmful reaction to the dye.

Limit yourself to clear liquids only for six to eight hours before the test. Arrange for someone to take you home a few hours after the test.

What to expect. About a half hour before the test, the doctor will give you a sedative and a painkiller. He'll also attach an intravenous line to your arm to make sure you don't become dehydrated, identify where the catheter will be inserted, and inject the anesthetic. Then he'll make a small incision and insert a thin catheter. Using a fluoro-scope — a machine that allows moving X-rays — the doctor guides the catheter into a major artery and toward the area he needs to examine. The doctor adds contrast dye through the catheter, which makes the X-rays easier to read. This might burn a little when he does this. While the doctor examines the arteries, still pictures called angiograms are taken.

Side effects and risks. Around 10 percent of the people who take this test have nausea or vomiting in reaction to the dye when it is injected. Other risks include radiation exposure, perforation of an artery, nerve injury, kidney failure as a reaction to the dye, bleeding where the catheter was inserted, or blood clots. Other rarer complications include heart attack, irregular heartbeats, and infection from arterial puncture.

After the test. Once the catheter is removed and the bleeding stopped, you must stay in bed with your legs straight for about four hours. To prevent bleeding, a small sandbag is often placed over your incision for a few hours. You will be encouraged to drink apple juice, water, or other clear fluids. Drink as much as you can to help flush the dye out of your body.

After a few hours, the area where the catheter was inserted is checked for bleeding or swelling. If everything looks normal, you'll be allowed to sit, stand, and walk for about 30 minutes. If there is no bleeding after that, someone can take you home. Before you go home, a doctor or nurse will show you how to stop any bleeding that may happen. Call for emergency medical help if bleeding lasts more than a few minutes. If the incision was made in your leg, don't overexert that leg for a few days.

Word to the wise

Abdominal angiography can also help deliver drugs directly into liver tumors or plug the source of intestinal bleeding with an artificial clot.

Advantages and disadvantages. This test gives your doctor a good look at the arteries in your abdominal organs. This test is invasive and includes risks like bleeding, clotting, allergic reaction to the dye, and radiation exposure. On a scale of 1 to 7 where 7 is the most expensive, this test rates a 5.

Fine needle biopsies

This test can help diagnose diseases in organs that can't be reached by endoscopy, like the liver and pancreas.

Before the test. Avoid food and drink for at least 12 hours before the test. Tell your doctor if you take an anticoagulant (blood thinner) or aspirin. These drugs can increase your risk of bleeding.

What to expect. While you lie on a table, the doctor will give you a shot of local anesthetic in the area where the biopsy will be done. Ultrasound or a CT scan may be used to help him guide the biopsy needle to the correct place. He'll use suction to draw out the tissue sample, which will take about one second. If several samples are needed, the needle will be inserted at several sites.

After the test. You'll stay in a recovery area for awhile so you can be monitored for signs of trouble. If your biopsy was a liver biopsy, you must lie on your right side for the first two hours, then stay in bed for 24 hours. Don't go back to your normal diet right away. Instead, drink only clear liquids for the first few hours. Then branch out to other liquids for 12 to 24 hours. You may have pain in your right shoulder for one to two days following the procedure.

Risks and side effects. Complications are rare but may include bleeding, bile leakage, and accidental injury to internal organs or blood vessels.

Advantages and disadvantages. Although it may mean you avoid endoscopy or some types of surgery, this test is invasive. The biopsy also provides less tissue than biopsy done during surgery, so the chances of a false negative are higher. You may still need exploratory surgery. On a cost scale of 1 to 7 where 7 is the most expensive, this test is a 3.

Index